bhakti-yoga

The Art of Eternal Love

ISKCON Silicon Valley
951 S Bascom Ave
San Jose, CA 95128
408-641-0197
www.virtualtemple.org

BOOKS by
His Divine Grace A. C. Bhaktivedanta Swami Prabhupāda

Bhagavad-gītā As It Is
Śrīmad-Bhāgavatam (completed by disciples)
Śrī Caitanya-caritāmṛta
Kṛṣṇa, the Supreme Personality of Godhead
Teachings of Lord Caitanya
The Nectar of Devotion
The Nectar of Instruction
Śrī Īśopaniṣad
Light of the Bhāgavata
Easy Journey to Other Planets
Teachings of Lord Kapila, the Son of Devahūti
Teachings of Queen Kuntī
Message of Godhead
The Science of Self-Realization
The Perfection of Yoga
Beyond Birth and Death
On the Way to Kṛṣṇa
Rāja-vidyā: The King of Knowledge
Elevation to Kṛṣṇa Consciousness
Kṛṣṇa Consciousness: The Matchless Gift
Kṛṣṇa Consciousness: The Topmost Yoga System
Perfect Questions, Perfect Answers
Life Comes from Life
The Nārada-bhakti-sūtra (completed by disciples)
The Mukunda-mālā-stotra (completed by disciples)
Geetār-gān (Bengali)
Vairāgya-vidyā (Bengali)
Buddhi-yoga (Bengali)
Bhakti-ratna-boli (Bengali)
Back to Godhead magazine (founder)

BOOKS compiled from the teachings of His Divine Grace A. C. Bhaktivedanta Swami Prabhupāda after his lifetime

Search for Liberation
A Second Chance
The Journey of Self-Discovery
Civilization and Transcendence
The Laws of Nature
Renunciation Through Wisdom
The Quest for Enlightenment
Dharma, the Way of Transcendence
Beyond Illusion and Doubt
The Hare Kṛṣṇa Challenge
Spiritual Yoga
Bhakti-yoga: the Art of Eternal Love

bhakti-yoga

The Art of Eternal Love

HIS DIVINE GRACE
A. C. Bhaktivedanta Swami Prabhupāda
Founder-Ācārya of the International Society for Krishna Consciousness

THE BHAKTIVEDANTA BOOK TRUST
Los Angeles • Stockholm • Mumbai • Sydney

ON THE COVER: In Vṛndāvana, Lord Kṛṣṇa's supreme spiritual abode, He engages in eternal exchanges of love with His dearest devotees, the cowherd girls, headed by Śrīmatī Rādhārāṇī.

Readers interested in the subject matter of this book are invited by the International Society for Krishna Consciousness to correspond with its secretary.

Bhakti-yoga: The Art of Eternal Love was prepared from the introduction and first chapter of Śrīla Prabhupāda's translation of the *Bhakti-rasāmṛta-sindhu,* called *The Nectar of Devotion,* along with transcripts of lectures he gave on that book in 1972 and 1973 in Vṛndāvana, Bombay, and Calcutta.

International Society for Krishna Consciousness
P.O. Box 341445
Los Angeles, California 90034, USA
Telephone: 1-800-927-4152 (Inside USA); 1-310-837-5283 (Outside USA)
Fax: 1-310-837-1056
e-mail: bbt.usa@krishna.com; web: www.krishna.com

International Society for Krishna Consciousness
P.O. Box 380
Riverstone, NSW 2765, Australia
Telephone: +61-2-9627-6306; Fax: +61-2-9627-6052
e-mail: bbt.au@krishna.com

Design: Arcita Dāsa
Cover Painting: "Kṛṣṇa Meets the Gopīs for the Rāsa Dance,"
by Parīkṣit Dāsa

Previous printings: 150,000; Current Printing, 2010: 100,000

Printed in Singapore

ISBN 0-89213-331-7

CONTENTS

INTRODUCTION

Love is one of the words we use most and understand least. The problem is that there are many kinds of love. One of the distinctions we can make between different kinds of love has to do with time, duration—how long love lasts. Some love lasts a few days, some lasts a lifetime, and some lasts forever. Most lovers aspire for the latter, but in vain.

Love between bodies is bound to be temporary, because the lovers' bodies are temporary. Ah, but what about the soul? Will the lovers not meet in the eternal spiritual world, and there enjoy deathless love?

Perhaps. But the question is, "How do we get to the spiritual world?" That requires a special kind of love, the love between the individual soul and the Supreme Soul, God. Actually, we are caught in a web of temporary, unsatisfying loving relationships because we have forgotten how to love God. So the spiritual love between the individual soul and the Supreme Soul is the most important kind of love. It is the only love that is truly eternal. Actually, every other kind of love we experience is just a reflection of the original loving exchange between the individual soul and the Supreme Soul. This special love is called, in Sanskrit, *bhakti*. And the process for awakening that love is called *bhakti-yoga,* the art of eternal love.

Bhakti involves three things: the lover, the beloved, and the loving relationship. In *bhakti,* all three are eternal. The lover, the individual soul, is eternal; the beloved, the Supreme Soul, is eternal; and the loving relationship, *bhakti,* is also eternal.

In the sixteenth century, an extremely advanced expert in *bhakti-yoga* named Śrīla Rūpa Gosvāmī wrote a handbook on its theory and practice. He called his book *Bhakti-rasāmṛta-sindhu,* "The Ocean of the Nectar of Divine Love." For a long time its secrets remained locked in the ancient Sanskrit language.

Fortunately for us, a modern master of the knowledge and techniques of *bhakti-yoga,* His Divine Grace A. C. Bhaktivedanta Swami Prabhupāda (known popularly as Śrīla Prabhupāda, translated the book into English and began training his students in its mysteries. Śrīla Prabhupāda titled his translation *The Nectar of Devotion*.

Love, in its material manifestation, is usually associated with places—a city like Paris in the springtime, or a beach where one walked with one's beloved. In the same way, spiritual love is also associated with places. The highest such place is Vṛndāvana, an earthly manifestation of the eternal spiritual place where God enjoys loving pastimes with His eternal associates in the spiritual sky. In Vṛndāvana there are many temples, and one of them, the Rādhā-Dāmodara temple, is forever associated with Rūpa Gosvāmī because his physical form is interred there. A small memorial to him (called a *samādhi*) rises in one of the temple courtyards.

Before he came to America in 1965, Śrīla Prabhupāda lived in a quiet room in the Rādhā-Dāmodara temple, and through his window he could see and draw inspiration from the *samādhi* of Rūpa Gosvāmī. Seven years later, Śrīla Prabhupāda returned to the Rādhā-Dāmodara temple. And in the courtyard, near Rūpa Gosvāmī's *samādhi*, he gave for his disciples a series of lectures on *The Nectar of Devotion*. Selections from those lectures, full of deep spiritual insight into *bhakti,* have been interwoven with excerpts from *The Nectar of Devotion* to form the substance of this book.

We invite you to share in Rūpa Gosvāmī's teachings on *bhakti-yoga,* the art of eternal love, as they have come down to us from his foremost modern follower in disciplic succession. If we can learn to love God through *bhakti-yoga,* then we can learn to love everything and everyone else in the proper way, in the way that will bring us the most happiness, the best happiness, the happiness of eternal love.

—The Editors

What Is "The Nectar of Devotion"?

The Nectar of Devotion is a summary study of the *Bhakti-rasāmṛta-sindhu,* which was written in Sanskrit by Śrīla Rūpa Gosvāmī Prabhupāda. He was the chief of the Six Gosvāmīs, who were the direct disciples of Lord Caitanya Mahāprabhu. When he first met Lord Caitanya, Śrīla Rūpa Gosvāmī Prabhupāda was engaged as a minister in the Muslim government of Bengal, India. He and his brother Sanātana were then named Dabira Khāsa and Sākara Mallika, respectively, and they held responsible posts as ministers of Nawab Hussain Shah. At that time, five hundred years ago, the Hindu society was very rigid, and if a member of the *brāhmaṇa* caste accepted a position of service under a Muslim ruler he was at once rejected from *brāhmaṇa* society. That was the position of the two brothers, Dabira Khāsa and Sākara Mallika. They belonged to the highly situated *sārasvata-brāhmaṇa* community, but they were ostracized due to their acceptance of ministerial posts in the government of Hussain Shah. It is the grace of Lord Caitanya that He accepted these two exalted personalities as His disciples and raised them to the position of *gosvāmīs,* the highest position of brahminical culture. Similarly, Lord Caitanya accepted Haridāsa Ṭhākura as His disciple, although Haridāsa happened to be born of a Muslim family, and Lord Caitanya later on made him the *ācārya* of the chanting of the holy name of the Lord: Hare Kṛṣṇa, Hare Kṛṣṇa, Kṛṣṇa Kṛṣṇa, Hare Hare/ Hare Rāma, Hare Rāma, Rāma Rāma, Hare Hare.

Lord Caitanya's principle is universal. Anyone who knows the science of Kṛṣṇa consciousness and is engaged in the service of the Lord is accepted as being in a higher position than a person born in the family of a *brāhmaṇa.* That is the original principle accepted by all Vedic literatures, especially by the *Bhagavad-gītā* and *Śrīmad-Bhāgavatam.* The principle of Lord Caitanya's movement in educating and elevating everyone to the exalted post of a *gosvāmī* is taught in *The Nectar of Devotion.*

Lord Caitanya met the two brothers Dabira Khāsa and Sākara Mallika in a village known as Rāmakeli, in the district of Maldah, and after that meeting the brothers decided to retire from government service and join Lord Caitanya. Dabira Khāsa, who was later to become Rūpa Gosvāmī, retired from his post and collected all the money he had accumulated during his service. It is described in the *Caitanya-caritāmṛta* that his accumulated savings in gold coins equaled millions of dollars and filled a large boat. He divided the money in a very exemplary manner, which should be followed by devotees in particular and by humanity in general. Fifty percent of his accumulated wealth was distributed to the Kṛṣṇa conscious persons, namely the *brāhmaṇas* and the Vaiṣṇavas; twenty-five percent was distributed to relatives; and twenty-five percent was kept against emergency expenditures and personal difficulties. Later on, when Sākara Mallika also proposed to retire, the Nawab was very much agitated and put him into jail. But Sākara Mallika, who was later to become Śrīla Sanātana Gosvāmī, took advantage of his brother's personal money, which had been deposited with a village banker, and escaped from the prison of Hussain Shah. In this way both brothers joined Lord Caitanya Mahāprabhu.

Rūpa Gosvāmī later met Lord Caitanya at Prayāga (Allahabad, India), and on the Daśāśvamedha bathing *ghāṭa* of that holy city the Lord instructed him continually for ten days. The Lord particularly instructed Rūpa Gosvāmī on the science of Kṛṣṇa consciousness. These teachings of Lord Caitanya to Śrīla Rūpa Gosvāmī Prabhupāda are narrated in our book *Teachings of Lord Caitanya.*

Later, Śrīla Rūpa Gosvāmī Prabhupāda elaborated the teachings of the Lord with profound knowledge of revealed scriptures and authoritative references from various Vedic literatures. Śrīla Śrīnivāsa Ācārya describes in his prayers to the Six Gosvāmīs that they were all highly learned scholars, not only in Sanskrit but also in foreign languages such as Persian and Arabic. They very scrutinizingly studied all the Vedic scriptures in order to establish the movement of Caitanya Mahāprabhu on the authorized principles of Vedic knowledge. The present Kṛṣṇa consciousness movement is also based on the authority of Śrīla Rūpa Gosvāmī Prabhupāda. We are therefore generally known as *rūpānugas,* or followers in the footsteps of Śrīla Rūpa Gosvāmī Prabhupāda. It is only for our guidance that Śrīla Rūpa Gosvāmī prepared his book *Bhakti-rasāmṛta-sindhu,* which is now presented in the form of *The Nectar of Devotion.*

What is Bhakti?

Bhakti means "devotional service." Every service has some attractive feature that drives the servitor progressively on and on. Every one of us within this world is perpetually engaged in some sort of service, and the impetus for such service is the pleasure we derive from it. Driven by affection for his wife and children, a family man works day and night. A philanthropist works in the same way for love of the greater family, and a nationalist for the cause of his country and countrymen. That force which drives the philanthropist, the householder, and the nationalist is called *rasa,* or a kind of mellow (relationship) whose taste is very sweet.

Bhakti-rasa is a mellow different from the ordinary *rasa* enjoyed by mundane workers. Mundane workers labor very hard day and night in order to relish a certain kind of *rasa* that is understood as sense gratification. The relish or taste of the mundane *rasa* does not long endure, and therefore mundane workers are always apt to change their position of enjoyment. A businessman is not satisfied by working the whole week; therefore, wanting a change for the weekend, he goes to a place where he tries to forget his business activities. Then, after the weekend is spent in forgetfulness, he again changes his position and resumes his actual business activities. Material engagement means accepting a particular status for some time and then changing it. This position of changing back and forth is technically known as *bhoga-tyāga,* which means a position of alternating sense enjoyment and renunciation.

A living entity cannot steadily remain either in sense enjoyment or in renunciation. Change is going on perpetually, and we cannot be happy in either state, because of our eternal constitutional position. Sense gratification does not endure for long, and it is therefore called *capala-sukha,* or flickering happiness. For example, an ordinary family man who works very hard day and night and is successful in giving comforts to the members of his family thereby relishes a kind of mellow, but his whole advancement of material happiness immediately terminates along with his body as soon as his life is over. Death is therefore taken as the representative of God for the atheistic class of men. The devotee realizes the presence of God by devotional service, whereas the atheist realizes the presence of God in the shape of death. At death everything is finished, and one has to begin a new chapter of life in a new situation, perhaps higher or lower than the last one. In any field of activity—political, social, national, or international—the result of our actions will be finished with the end of life. That is sure.

Bhakti-rasa, however, the mellow relished in the transcendental loving service of the Lord, does not finish with the end of life. It continues perpetually and is therefore called *amṛta,* that which does not die but exists eternally. This is confirmed in all Vedic literatures. The *Bhagavad-gītā* says that a little advancement in *bhakti-rasa* can save the devotee from the greatest danger—that of missing the opportunity to be a human being in the next life. The *rasas* derived from our feelings in social life, in family life, or in the greater family life of altruism, philanthropy, nationalism, socialism, communism, etc., do not guarantee that one's next life will be as a human being. We prepare our next life by our actual activities in the present life. A living entity is offered a particular type of body as a result of his action in the present body. These activities are taken into account by a superior authority known as *daiva,* or the authority of God. This *daiva* is explained in the *Bhagavad-gītā* as the prime cause of everything, and in *Śrīmad-Bhāgavatam* it is stated that a man takes his next body by *daiva-netreṇa,* which means by the supervision of the authority of the Supreme. In an ordinary sense, *daiva* is explained as "destiny." *Daiva* supervision gives us a body selected from 8,400,000 forms; the choice does not depend on our selection, but is awarded to us according to our destiny. If our body at present is engaged in the activities of Kṛṣṇa consciousness, then it is guaranteed that we will have at least a human body in our next life. A human being engaged in Kṛṣṇa consciousness, even if unable to complete the course of *bhakti-yoga,* takes birth in the higher divisions of human society so that he can automatically further his advancement in Kṛṣṇa consciousness. Therefore, all bona fide activities in Kṛṣṇa consciousness are *amṛta,* or permanent. This is the subject matter of *The Nectar of Devotion.*

Benefits of Bhakti

This eternal engagement in *bhakti-rasa* can be understood by a serious student upon studying *The Nectar of Devotion.* Adoption of *bhakti-rasa,* or Kṛṣṇa consciousness, will immediately bring one to an auspicious life free from anxieties and will bless one with transcendental existence, thus minimizing the value of liberation. *Bhakti-rasa* itself is sufficient to produce a feeling of liberation, because it attracts the attention of the Supreme Lord, Kṛṣṇa. Generally, neophyte devotees are anxious to see Kṛṣṇa, or God, but God cannot be seen or known by our present materially blunt senses. The process of devotional service as it is recommended in *The Nectar of Devotion* will gradually elevate one from the material condition of life to the spiritual status, wherein the devotee becomes purified of all designations. The senses can then become uncontaminated, being constantly in touch with *bhakti-rasa.* When the purified senses are employed in the service of the Lord, one becomes situated in *bhakti-rasa* life, and any action performed for the satisfaction of Kṛṣṇa in this transcendental *bhakti-rasa* stage of life can be relished perpetually. When one is thus engaged in devotional service, all varieties of *rasas,* or mellows, turn into eternity. In the beginning one is trained according to the principles of regulation under the guidance of the *ācārya,* or spiritual master, and gradually, when one is elevated, devotional service becomes automatic and spontaneous eagerness to serve Kṛṣṇa. There are twelve kinds of *rasas,* which are explained in *The Nectar of Devotion,* and by renovating our relationship with Kṛṣṇa in five primary *rasas* we can live eternally in full knowledge and bliss.

The basic principle of the living condition is that we have a general propensity to love someone. No one can live without loving someone else. This propensity is present in every living being. Even an animal like a tiger has this loving propensity at least in a dormant stage, and it is certainly present in the human beings. The missing point, however, is where to repose our love so that everyone can become happy. At the present moment the human society teaches one to love his country or family or his personal self, but there is no information where to repose the loving propensity so that everyone can become happy. That missing point is Kṛṣṇa, and *The Nectar of Devotion* teaches us how to stimulate our original love for Kṛṣṇa and how to be situated in that position where we can enjoy our blissful life.

In the primary stage a child loves his parents, then his brothers and sisters, and as he daily grows up he begins to love his family, society, community, country, nation, or even the whole human society. But the loving propensity is not satisfied even by loving all human society; that loving propensity remains imperfectly fulfilled until we know who is the supreme beloved. Our love can be fully satisfied only when it is reposed in Kṛṣṇa. This theme is the sum and substance of *The Nectar of Devotion,* which teaches us how to love Kṛṣṇa in five different transcendental mellows.

Boundless Love

Our loving propensity expands just as a vibration of light or air expands, but we do not know where it ends. *The Nectar of Devotion* teaches us the science of loving every one of the living entities perfectly by the easy method of loving Kṛṣṇa. We have failed to create peace and harmony in human society, even by such great attempts as the United Nations, because we do not know the right method. The method is very simple, but one has to understand it with a cool head. *The Nectar of Devotion* teaches all men how to perform the simple and natural method of loving Kṛṣṇa, the Supreme Personality of Godhead. If we learn how to love Kṛṣṇa, then it is very easy to immediately and simultaneously love every living being. It is like pouring water on the root of a tree or supplying food to one's stomach. The method of pouring water on the root of a tree or supplying food to the stomach is universally scientific and practical, as every one of us has experienced. Everyone knows well that when we eat something, or in other words, when we put food into the stomach, the energy created by such action is immediately distributed throughout the whole body. Similarly, when we pour water on the root, the energy thus created is immediately distributed throughout the entirety of even the largest tree. It is not possible to water the tree part by part, nor is it possible to feed the different parts of the body separately. *The Nectar of Devotion* will teach us how to turn the one switch that will immediately brighten everything, everywhere. One who does not know this method is missing the point of life.

As far as material necessities are concerned, the human civilization at the present moment is very much advanced in living comfortably, but still we are not happy, because we are missing the point. The material comforts of life alone are not sufficient to make us happy. The root cause of our dissatisfaction is that our dormant loving propensity has not been fulfilled despite our great advancement in the materialistic way of life. *The Nectar of Devotion* will give us practical hints how we can live in this material world perfectly engaged in devotional service and thus fulfill all our desires in this life and the next.

The Nectar of Devotion is not presented to condemn any way of materialistic life, but the attempt is to give information to religionists, philosophers, and people in general how to love Kṛṣṇa. One may live without material discomfiture, but at the same time one should learn the art of loving Kṛṣṇa. At the present moment we are inventing so many ways to utilize our propensity to love, but factually we are missing the real point: Kṛṣṇa. We are watering all parts of the tree, but missing the tree's root. We are trying to keep our body fit by all means, but we are neglecting to supply food to the stomach. Missing Kṛṣṇa means missing one's self also. Real self-realization and realization of Kṛṣṇa go together simultaneously. For example, seeing oneself in the morning means seeing the sunrise also; without seeing the sunshine no one can see himself. Similarly, unless one has realized Kṛṣṇa there is no question of self-realization.

Definition of Pure Devotional Service

The authorized descriptions of *bhakti,* or devotional service, following in the footsteps of previous *ācāryas,* can be summarized in the following statement by Śrīla Rūpa Gosvāmī: "First-class devotional service is known by one's tendency to be fully engaged in Kṛṣṇa consciousness, serving the Lord favorably." The purport is that one may also be in Kṛṣṇa consciousness unfavorably, but that cannot be counted as pure devotional service. Pure devotional service should be free from the desire for any material benefit or for sense gratification, as these desires are cultivated through fruitive activities and philosophical speculation. Generally, people are engaged in different activities to get some material profit, while most philosophers are engaged in proposing transcendental realization through volumes of word jugglery and speculation. Pure devotional service must always be free from such fruitive activities and philosophical speculations. One has to learn Kṛṣṇa consciousness, or pure devotional service, from the authorities by spontaneous loving service.

Acting for Kṛṣṇa: The Essence of Bhakti

This devotional service is a sort of cultivation. It is not simply inaction for people who like to be inactive or devote their time to silent meditation. There are many different methods for people who want this, but cultivation of Kṛṣṇa consciousness is different. The particular word used by Śrīla Rūpa Gosvāmī in this connection is *anuśīlana,* or cultivation by following the predecessor teachers (*ācāryas*). As soon as we say "cultivation," we must refer to activity. Without activity, consciousness alone cannot help us. All activities may be divided into two classes: one class may be for achieving a certain goal, and the other may be for avoiding some unfavorable circumstance. In Sanskrit, these activities are called *pravṛtti* and *nivṛtti*—positive and negative action. There are many examples of negative action. For instance, a diseased person has to be cautious and take medicine in order to avoid making his illness worse.

Those who are cultivating spiritual life and executing devotional service are always engaged in activity. Such activity can be performed with the body or with the mind. Thinking, feeling, and willing are all activities of the mind, and when we will to do something, the activity comes to be manifest by the gross bodily senses. Thus, in our mental activities we should always try to think of Kṛṣṇa and try to plan how to please Him, following in the footsteps of the great *ācāryas* and the personal spiritual master. There are activities of the body, activities of the mind, and activities of speech. A Kṛṣṇa conscious person engages his words in preaching the glories of the Lord. This is called *kīrtana.* And by his mind a Kṛṣṇa conscious person always thinks of the activities of the Lord—as He is speaking on the Battlefield of Kurukṣetra or engaging in His various pastimes in Vṛndāvana with His devotees. In this way one can always think of the activities and pastimes of the Lord. This is the mental culture of Kṛṣṇa consciousness.

Similarly, we can offer many services with our bodily activities. But all such activities must be in relationship with Kṛṣṇa. This relationship is established by connecting oneself with the bona fide spiritual master, who is the direct representative of Kṛṣṇa in disciplic succession. Therefore, the execution of Kṛṣṇa conscious activities with the body should be directed by the spiritual master and then performed with faith. The connection with the spiritual master is called initiation. From the date of initiation by the spiritual master, the connection between Kṛṣṇa and a person cultivating Kṛṣṇa consciousness is established. Without initiation by a bona fide spiritual master, the actual connection with Kṛṣṇa consciousness is never performed.

This cultivation of Kṛṣṇa consciousness is not material. The Lord has three general energies—namely the external energy, the internal energy, and the marginal energy. The living entities are called marginal energy, and the material cosmic manifestation is the action of the external, or material, energy. Then there is the spiritual world, which is a manifestation of the internal energy. The living entities, who are called marginal energy, perform material activities when acting under the inferior, external energy. And when they engage in activities under the internal, spiritual energy, their activities are called Kṛṣṇa conscious. This means that those who are great souls or great devotees do not act under the spell of the material energy, but act instead under the protection of the spiritual energy. Any activities done in devotional service, or in Kṛṣṇa consciousness, are directly under the control of the spiritual energy. In other words, energy is a sort of strength, and this strength can be spiritualized by the mercy of both the bona fide spiritual master and Kṛṣṇa.

In the *Caitanya-caritāmṛta,* by Kṛṣṇadāsa Kavirāja Gosvāmī, Lord Caitanya states that it is a fortunate person who comes in contact with a bona fide spiritual master by the grace of Kṛṣṇa. To one who is serious about spiritual life Kṛṣṇa gives the intelligence to come in contact with a bona fide spiritual master, and then by the grace of the spiritual master one becomes advanced in Kṛṣṇa consciousness. In this way the whole jurisdiction of Kṛṣṇa consciousness is directly under the spiritual energy—Kṛṣṇa and the spiritual master.

Definition of A Pure Devotee

The definition of a pure devotee, as given by Rūpa Gosvāmī in his *Bhakti-rasāmṛta-sindhu,* can be summarized thus: his service is favorable and is always in relation to Kṛṣṇa. In order to keep the purity of such Kṛṣṇa conscious activities, one must be freed from all material desires and philosophical speculation. Any desire except for the service of the Lord is called material desire. And "philosophical speculation" refers to the sort of speculation which ultimately arrives at a conclusion of voidism or impersonalism. This conclusion is useless for a Kṛṣṇa conscious person. Only rarely by philosophical speculation can one reach the conclusion of worshiping Vāsudeva, or Kṛṣṇa. This is confirmed in the *Bhagavad-gītā* itself. The ultimate end of philosophical speculation, then, must be Kṛṣṇa, with the understanding that Kṛṣṇa is everything, the cause of all causes, and that one should therefore surrender unto Him. If this ultimate goal is reached, then philosophical advancement is favorable, but if the conclusion of philosophical speculation is voidism or impersonalism, that is not *bhakti.*

Karma, or fruitive activities, is sometimes understood to consist of ritualistic activities. There are many persons who are very much attracted by the ritualistic activities described in the

Vedas. But if one becomes attracted simply to ritualistic activities without understanding Kṛṣṇa, his activities are unfavorable to Kṛṣṇa consciousness. Actually, Kṛṣṇa consciousness can be based simply on hearing about Kṛṣṇa, chanting about Him, remembering Him, etc. The *Śrīmad-Bhāgavatam* describes nine different processes, besides which everything done is unfavorable to Kṛṣṇa consciousness.

Śrīla Rūpa Gosvāmī has also quoted a definition from the *Nārada-pañcarātra,* as follows: "One should be free from all material designations and, by Kṛṣṇa consciousness, must be cleansed of all material contamination. He should be restored to his pure identity, in which he engages his senses in the service of the proprietor of the senses." So when our senses are engaged for Kṛṣṇa, the actual proprietor of the senses, that activity is called devotional service. In our conditioned state our senses are engaged in serving the bodily demands. When the same senses are engaged in executing the order of Kṛṣṇa, our activities are called *bhakti.*

As long as one identifies himself as belonging to a certain family, a certain society, or a certain nation, he is said to be covered with designations. When one is fully aware that he does not belong to any family, society, or country but is eternally related to Kṛṣṇa, he then realizes that his energy should be employed not in the interests of so-called family, society, or country but in the interests of Kṛṣṇa. This is purity of purpose and the platform of pure devotional service in Kṛṣṇa consciousness.

Six Features of Pure Bhakti

Next Rūpa Gosvāmī gives six unique features of pure devotional service.

(1) Pure devotional service brings immediate relief from all kinds of material distress.

(2) Pure devotional service is the beginning of all auspiciousness.

(3) Pure devotional service automatically puts one in transcendental pleasure.

(4) Pure devotional service is rarely achieved.

(5) Those in pure devotional service deride even the conception of liberation.

(6) Pure devotional service is the only means to attract Kṛṣṇa. Kṛṣṇa is all-attractive, but pure devotional service attracts even Him. This means that pure devotional service is even transcendentally stronger than Kṛṣṇa Himself, because it is Kṛṣṇa's internal potency.

(1)
Kṛṣṇa Consciousness Brings Relief from All Material Distress

In the *Bhagavad-gītā,* the Lord says that one should surrender unto Him, giving up all other engagements. The Lord also gives His word there that He will protect surrendered souls from the reactions of all sinful activities. Śrīla Rūpa Gosvāmī says that the distresses from sinful activities are due both to the sins themselves and to sins committed in our past lives. Generally, one commits sinful activities due to ignorance. But ignorance is no excuse for evading the reaction—distresses. Sinful activities are of two kinds: those which are mature and those which are not mature. The sinful activities for which we are suffering at the present moment are called mature. The many sinful activities stored within us for which we have not yet suffered are considered immature. For example, a man may have committed criminal acts but not yet been arrested for them. Now, as soon as he is detected, arrest is awaiting him. Similarly, for some of our sinful activities we are awaiting distresses in the future, and for others, which are mature, we are suffering at the present moment.

In this way there is a chain of sinful activities and their concomitant distresses, and the conditioned soul is suffering life after life due to these sins. He is suffering in the present life the results of sinful activities from his past life, and he is meanwhile creating further sufferings for his future life. Mature sinful activities are exhibited if one is suffering from some chronic disease, if one is suffering from some legal implication, if one is born in a low and degraded family, or if one is uneducated or very ugly.

There are many results of past sinful activities for which we are suffering at the present moment, and we may be suffering in the future due to our present sinful activities. But all of these reactions to sinful deeds can immediately be stopped if we take to Kṛṣṇa consciousness. As evidence for this, Rūpa Gosvāmī quotes a verse from the *Śrīmad-Bhāgavatam* (11.14.19). This verse is in connection with Lord Kṛṣṇa's instruction to Uddhava, where He says, "My dear Uddhava, devotional service unto Me is just like a blazing fire that can burn into ashes unlimited fuel supplied to it." The purport is that as the blazing fire can burn any amount of fuel to ashes, so devotional service to the Lord in Kṛṣṇa consciousness can burn up all the fuel of sinful activities. For example, in the *Gītā* Arjuna thought that fighting was a sinful activity, but Kṛṣṇa engaged him on the battlefield under His order, and so the fighting became devotional service. Therefore, Arjuna was not subjected to any sinful reaction.

Śrīla Rūpa Gosvāmī quotes a verse from the Third Canto of *Śrīmad-Bhāgavatam* (3.33.6), in which Devahūti addresses her son, Kapiladeva, an incarnation of Kṛṣṇa who taught a type of yoga called *sāṅkhya,* and says, "My dear Lord, there are nine different kinds of devotional service, beginning from hearing and chanting. Anyone who hears about Your pastimes, who chants about Your glories, who offers You obeisances, who thinks of You and, in this way, executes any of the nine kinds of devotional service—even if he is born in a family of dog-eaters [the lowest grade of mankind]—becomes immediately qualified to perform sacrifices." As such, how is it possible that anyone actually engaged in devotional service in full Kṛṣṇa consciousness has not become purified? It is not possible. One who is engaged in Kṛṣṇa consciousness and devotional service has without doubt become freed from all contaminations of material sinful activities. Devotional service therefore has the power to actually nullify all kinds of reactions to sinful deeds. A devotee is nevertheless always alert not to commit any sinful activities; this is his specific qualification as a devotee. Thus the *Śrīmad-Bhāgavatam* states that by performing devotional service a person who was born even in a family of dog-eaters may become eligible to take part in the performance of the ritualistic ceremonies recommended in the *Vedas.* It is implicit in this statement that a person born into a family of dog-eaters is generally not fit for performing *yajña,* or sacrifice. The priestly caste in charge of performing these ritualistic ceremonies recommended in the *Vedas* is called the *brāhmaṇa* order. Unless one is a *brāhmaṇa,* he cannot perform these ceremonies.

A person is born in a *brāhmaṇa* family or in a family of dog-eaters due to his past activities. If a person is born in a family of dog-eaters it means that his past activities were all sinful. But if even such a person takes to the path of devotional service and begins to chant the holy names of the Lord—Hare Kṛṣṇa, Hare Kṛṣṇa, Kṛṣṇa Kṛṣṇa, Hare Hare/ Hare Rāma, Hare Rāma, Rāma Rāma, Hare Hare—he is at once fit to perform the ritualistic ceremonies. This means that his sinful reactions have immediately become neutralized.

It is stated in the *Padma Purāṇa* that there are four kinds of effects due to sinful activities, which are listed as follows: (1) the effect which is not yet fructified, (2) the effect which is lying as seed, (3) the effect which is already mature and (4) the effect which is almost mature. It is also stated that all these four effects become immediately vanquished for those who surrender unto the Supreme Personality of Godhead, Viṣṇu, and become engaged in His devotional service in full Kṛṣṇa consciousness.

Those effects described as "almost mature" refer to the distress from which one is suffering at present, and the effects "lying as seed" are in the core of the heart, where there is a certain stock of sinful desires, which are like seeds. The Sanskrit word *kūṭam* means that they are almost ready to produce the seed, or the effect of the seed. "An immature effect" refers to the case where the seedling has not begun. From this statement of *Padma Purāṇa* it is understood that material contamination is very subtle. Its beginning, its fruition and results, and how one suffers such results in the form of distress, are part of a great chain. When one catches some disease, it is often very difficult to ascertain the cause of the disease, where it originated, and how it is maturing. The suffering of a disease, however, does not appear all of a sudden. It actually takes time. And as in the medical field, for precaution's sake, the doctor injects a vaccination to prevent the growing of contamination, the practical injection to stop all the fructifications of the seeds of our sinful activities is simply engagement in Kṛṣṇa consciousness.

Ajāmila, a Sinner Saved

In this connection, Śukadeva Gosvāmī speaks in the Sixth Canto of *Śrīmad-Bhāgavatam* (6.2.17) about the story of Ajāmila, who began life as a fine and dutiful *brāhmaṇa* but who in his young manhood became wholly corrupted by a prostitute. At the end of his wicked life, just by calling the name "Nārāyaṇa [Kṛṣṇa]," he was saved despite so much sin. Śukadeva points out that austerity, charity, and the performance of ritualistic ceremonies for counteracting sinful activities are recommended processes, but that by performing them one cannot remove the sinful desire-seed from the heart, as was the case with Ajāmila in his youth. This sinful desire-seed can be removed only by achieving Kṛṣṇa consciousness. And this can be accomplished very easily by chanting the *mahā-mantra,* or Hare Kṛṣṇa *mantra,* as recommended by Śrī Caitanya Mahāprabhu. In other words, unless one adopts the path of devotional service, one cannot be one-hundred-percent clean from all sinful reactions .

By performing Vedic ritualistic activities, by giving money in charity, and by undergoing austerity one can temporarily become free from the reactions of sinful activities, but at the next moment one must again become engaged in sinful activities. For example, a person suffering from venereal disease on account of excessive indulgence in sex life has to undergo some severe pain in medical treatment, and he is then cured for the time being. But because he has not been able to remove the sex desire from his heart, he must again indulge in the same thing and become a victim of the same disease. So medical treatment may give temporary relief from the distress of such venereal disease, but unless one is trained to understand that sex life is abominable, it is impossible to be saved from such repeated distress. Similarly, the ritualistic performances, charity, and austerity that are recommended in the *Vedas* may temporarily stop one from acting in sinful ways, but as long as the heart is not clear, one will have to repeat sinful activities again and again.

Another example given in the *Śrīmad-Bhāgavatam* concerns the elephant who enters a lake and takes a bath very seriously, cleansing his body thoroughly. Then as soon as he comes onto the shore he again takes some dust from the earth and throws it over his body. Similarly, a person who is not trained in Kṛṣṇa consciousness cannot become completely free from the desire for sinful activities. Neither the meditative yoga process nor philosophical speculations nor fruitive activities can save one from the seeds of sinful desires. Only by being engaged in devotional service can this be done.

There is another evidence in the Fourth Canto of *Śrīmad-Bhāgavatam* (4.22.39), wherein Sanat-kumāra says, "My dear king, the false ego of a human being is so strong that it keeps him in material existence as if tied up by a strong rope. Only the devotees can cut off the knot of this strong rope very easily, by engaging themselves in Kṛṣṇa consciousness. Others, who are not in Kṛṣṇa consciousness but are trying to become great mystics or great ritual performers, cannot advance like the devotees.

Therefore, it is the duty of everyone to engage himself in the activities of Kṛṣṇa consciousness in order to be freed from the tight knot of false ego and engagement in material activities."

This tight knot of false ego is due to ignorance. As long as one is ignorant about his identity, he is sure to act wrongly and thereby become entangled in material contamination. This ignorance of factual knowledge can also be dissipated by Kṛṣṇa consciousness, as is confirmed in the *Padma Purāṇa* as follows: "Pure devotional service in Kṛṣṇa consciousness is the highest enlightenment, and when such enlightenment is there, it is just like a blazing forest fire, killing all the inauspicious snakes of desire." The example is being given in this connection that when there is a forest fire the extensive blazing automatically kills all the snakes in the forest. There are many, many snakes on the ground of the forest, and when a fire takes place, it burns the dried foliage, and the snakes are immediately attacked. Animals who have four legs can flee from the fire or can at least try to flee, but the snakes are immediately killed. Similarly, the blazing fire of Kṛṣṇa consciousness is so strong that the snakes of ignorance are immediately killed.

Kṛṣṇa's Promise

Everyone in the material world is full of anxieties. That is the nature of material existence. One after another, problems come. So if someone would promise us, "Just depend on me; I will solve all your problems," how much relief we would feel! Just imagine! Of course, we may not believe it. If some ordinary human being says to us, "Do not worry; I will take charge of all your affairs," we may doubt his ability to do so because we know his limitations. But when Kṛṣṇa says, "I will take charge of you," we should have full faith in His words and feel so much relief. Kṛṣṇa is not an ordinary man—He is the all-powerful Supreme Personality of Godhead. He is Yogeśvara, the master of all mystic power, and He is the Absolute Truth. Therefore, when He promises in the *Bhagavad-gītā*, "Give up all other attempts to solve your prob-

The Cycle of Suffering

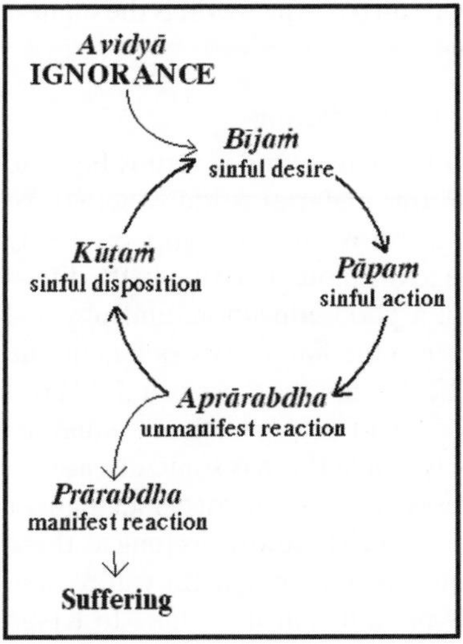

The root cause of suffering is avidyā, ignorance of our real identity as eternal servants of Lord Kṛṣṇa. Because of this ignorance, we tend to acquire sinful desires (bījam) in contact with the objects of the senses. When we act on these desires, we commit sin (pāpam). The sinful reaction is at first unmanifest (aprārabdha), but over time (even over lifetimes) the reaction to sin manifests as suffering (prārabdha) and the disposition to commit further sin (kūṭam). The process of bhakti, or Kṛṣṇa consciousness, counteracts all these stages of suffering.

lems and just surrender to Me. I will take charge of you and nullify all your sinful reactions," we should feel assured that we will be delivered from the reactions of all our sinful activities.

(2)
Kṛṣṇa Consciousness Is All-Auspicious

Śrīla Rūpa Gosvāmī has given a definition of auspiciousness. He says that actual auspiciousness means welfare activities for all the people of the world. At the present moment groups of people are engaged in welfare activities in terms of society, community, or nation. There is even an attempt in the form of the United Nations for world-help activity. But due to the shortcomings of limited national activities, such a general mass welfare program for the whole world is not practically possible. The Kṛṣṇa consciousness movement, however, is so nice that it can render the highest benefit to the entire human race. Everyone can be attracted by this movement, and everyone can feel the result. Therefore, Rūpa Gosvāmī and other learned scholars agree that a broad propaganda program for the Kṛṣṇa consciousness movement of devotional service all over the world is the highest humanitarian welfare activity.

The End of All Suffering

We suffer because of our sinful activities, and we enjoy because of our pious activities. But in this material world, whether we enjoy or suffer, the common factor is suffering. Suppose in my next life I get a good birth due to my pious activities in this life—I may have sufficient wealth, a good education, and physical beauty. But even if I'm born into the family of a rich man, the sufferings of taking birth will be the same as those of a child born into a poor family. The sufferings of taking birth are equal for the poor and the rich. Similarly, when there is some disease—a fever, for example—it is not less painful for the rich man than for the poor man. The pain is the same. Therefore, as long as there is material existence, this suffering and enjoyment will remain on the same level: ultimately painful. But if we take to Kṛṣṇa consciousness, Kṛṣṇa assures us, *ahaṁ tvāṁ sarva-pāpebhyo mokṣayiṣyāmi:* "I will free you from all sins and all suffering." That is real auspiciousness.

When Kṛṣṇa takes charge of us, He gradually educates us from within and without so that we may go back home, back to Godhead. From the material point of view it is auspicious to achieve wealth, education, beauty, high parentage, and so on, but all these are adulterated with so many sufferings. Therefore, they are not actually auspicious. Real auspiciousness is to go back home, back to Godhead, for an eternal life of bliss and knowledge. And that can be achieved only by engagement in pure devotional service to Lord Kṛṣṇa, without any material motive. So engaging in pure devotional service is the beginning of all auspiciousness. And to achieve that we have to follow the rules and regulations, chant the Hare Kṛṣṇa *mahā-mantra* daily, and engage always in the service of the Lord.

(3)
Kṛṣṇa Consciousness Produces Supreme Happiness

Śrīla Rūpa Gosvāmī has analyzed the different sources of happiness. He has divided happiness into three categories, which are (1) happiness derived from material enjoyment, (2) happiness derived by identifying oneself with the Supreme Brahman, and (3) happiness derived from Kṛṣṇa consciousness.

In the *tantra-śāstra* Lord Śiva speaks to his wife, Satī, in this way: "My dear wife, a person who has surrendered himself at the lotus feet of Govinda and who has thus developed pure Kṛṣṇa consciousness can be very easily awarded all the perfections desired by the impersonalists; and beyond this, he can enjoy the happiness achieved by the pure devotees."

Happiness derived from pure devotional service is the highest because it is eternal, whereas the happiness derived from material perfection or from understanding oneself to be Brahman is inferior because it is temporary. There is no preventing one's falling down from material happiness, and there is even every chance of falling down from the spiritual happiness derived out of identifying oneself with the impersonal Brahman.

It has been seen that great Māyāvādī *sannyāsīs*—very highly educated and almost realized souls—may sometimes take to political activities or to social welfare activities. The reason is that they actually do not derive any ultimate transcendental happiness in the impersonal understanding and therefore must come down to the material platform and take to such mundane affairs. There are many instances, especially in India, where these Māyāvādī *sannyāsīs* descend to the material platform again. But a person who is fully in Kṛṣṇa consciousness will never return to any sort of material platform. However alluring and attractive they may be, he always knows that no material welfare activities can compare to the spiritual activity of Kṛṣṇa consciousness.

Happiness from Nondevotional Yoga Is Inferior

The mystic perfections achieved by actually successful yogis are eight in number. *Aṇimā-siddhi* refers to the power by which one can become so small that he can enter into a stone. But modern scientific improvements also enable us to enter into stone, because they provide for excavating so many subways, penetrating the hills, etc. So *aṇimā-siddhi,* the mystic perfection of trying to enter into stone, has also been achieved by material science. Similarly, all of the *yoga-siddhis,* or perfections, are material arts. For example, in one *yoga-siddhi* there is development of the power to become so light that one can float in the air or on water. That has also been achieved by modern science. It has enabled us to fly in the air, float on the surface of the water, and travel under the water.

Of course, in the categories of mystic perfection there are certain processes that the material scientists have not yet been able to develop. For instance, a mystic yogi can enter into the sun planet simply by using the rays of the sunshine. This perfection is called *laghimā.* Similarly, a yogi can touch the moon with his finger. Though the modern astronauts go to the moon with the help of spaceships, they undergo many difficulties, whereas a person with mystic perfection can extend his hand and touch the moon with his finger. This *siddhi* is called *prāpti,* or acquisition. With this *prāpti-siddhi,* not only can the perfect mystic yogi touch the moon planet, but he can extend his hand anywhere and take whatever he likes. He may be sitting thousands of miles away from a certain place, and if he likes he can take fruit from a garden there. This is *prāpti-siddhi.*

The modern scientists have manufactured nuclear weapons with which they can destroy an insignificant part of this planet, but by the *yoga-siddhi* known as *īśitā* one can create and destroy an entire planet simply at will. Another perfection is called *vaśitā,* and by this perfection one can bring anyone under his control. This is a kind of hypnotism that is almost irresistible. Sometimes it is found that a yogi who may have attained a little perfection in this *vaśitā* mystic power comes out among the people and speaks all sorts of nonsense, controls their minds, exploits them, takes their money, and then goes away.

There is another mystic perfection, which is known as *prākāmya* (magic). By this *prākāmya* power one can achieve anything he likes. For example, one can make water enter into his eye and then again come out from within the eye. Simply by his will he can perform such wonderful activities.

The highest perfection of mystic power is called *kāmāvasāyitā.* This is also magic, but whereas the *prākāmya* power acts to create wonderful effects within the scope of nature, *kāmāvasāyitā* permits one to contradict nature—in other words, to do the impossible. Of course, one can derive great amounts of temporary happiness by achieving such yogic materialistic perfections.

Material Happiness: Temporary at Best

Foolishly, people who are enamored of the glitter of modern materialistic advancement are thinking that the Kṛṣṇa consciousness movement is for less intelligent men. "I am better off being busy with my material comforts—maintaining a nice apartment, family, and sex life." These people do not know that at any moment they can be kicked out of their material situation. Due to ignorance, they do not know that real life is eternal. The temporary comforts of the body are not the goal of life, and it is due only to darkest ignorance that people become enamored of the glimmering advancement of material comforts. Śrīla Bhaktivinoda Ṭhākura has therefore said that the advancement of material knowledge renders a person more foolish, because it causes one to forget his real identity by its glitter. This is doom for him, because this human form of life is meant for getting out of material contamination. By the advancement of material knowledge, people are becoming more and more entangled in material existence. They have no hope of being liberated from this catastrophe.

Rejecting the Dream of Material Happiness

We are enamored by the glitter of this material world just as moths are attracted by a fire. Moths enter with great speed into the fire, without knowing that they are going to die. Their forceful entrance into the fire means sure death. Similarly, modern science has created some so-called comforts of life for temporary enjoyment, but at the same time we take the risk of so many dangerous conditions. As the *Śrīmad-Bhāgavatam* says, *padaṁ padaṁ yad vipadām:* In this world there is danger at every step.

Our attempts to mitigate discomfort are like the attempts of a laborer to get some relief when carrying a heavy burden. When he is too uncomfortable, he shifts the burden from his head to his shoulder. But that does not eliminate the difficulty of carrying the burden. Similarly, we are trying to get material comforts by producing so many scientific inventions, but they do not actually provide happiness. We are simply changing the position of our burden. For instance, in America the people have to accept so much danger just to drive around in their motorcars. They may try to increase their happiness by improving transportation, but they are just shifting the burden around. They therefore create more and more problems. They have so many cars that they have to construct more roads and highways, one on top of another. Still they experience traffic congestion, accidents, pollution, and discomfort. This is a vain endeavor. The scientists think they are solving the problems of life, but the discomforts of life are still there. And the scientists must fail, because this material world is by nature full of discomfort, as Kṛṣṇa Himself confirms in the *Bhagavad-gītā: duḥkhālayam aśāśvatam*. How, then, can you make it a happy place?

We may dream of something dangerous, that a tiger or snake is coming, and then we want to change to another dream. Similarly, our attempt to become happy in this material world by manufacturing some artificial means of happiness is simply a useless dream. Real happiness is to take shelter of the lotus feet of Kṛṣṇa.

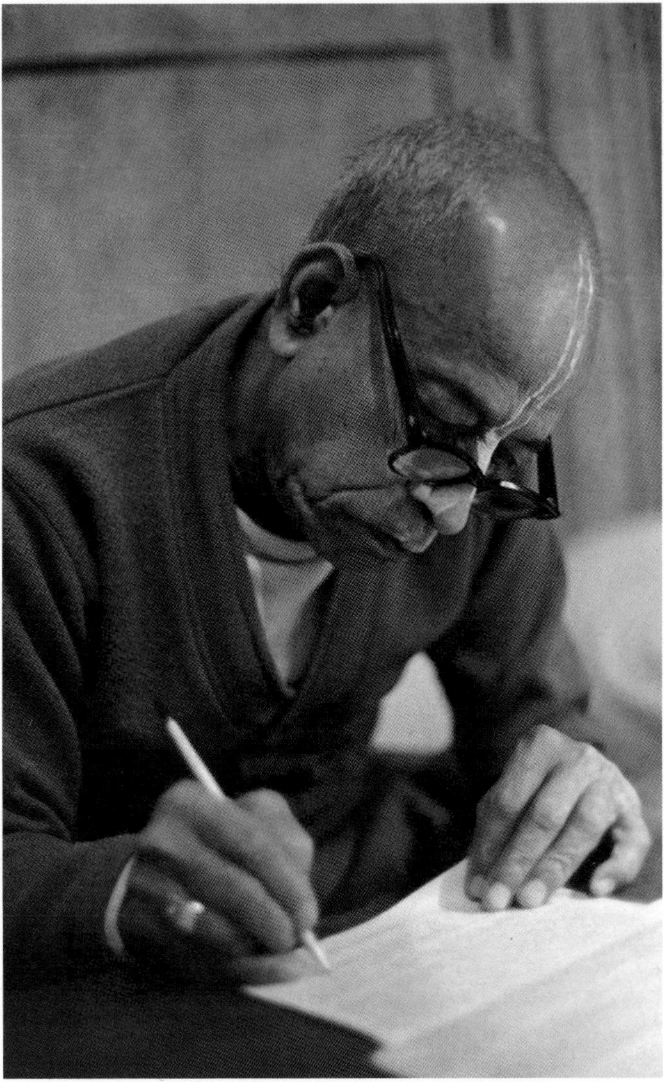

His Divine Grace
A. C. Bhaktivedanta Swami Prabhupāda
Founder-*ācārya* of the International Society for Krishna Consciousness

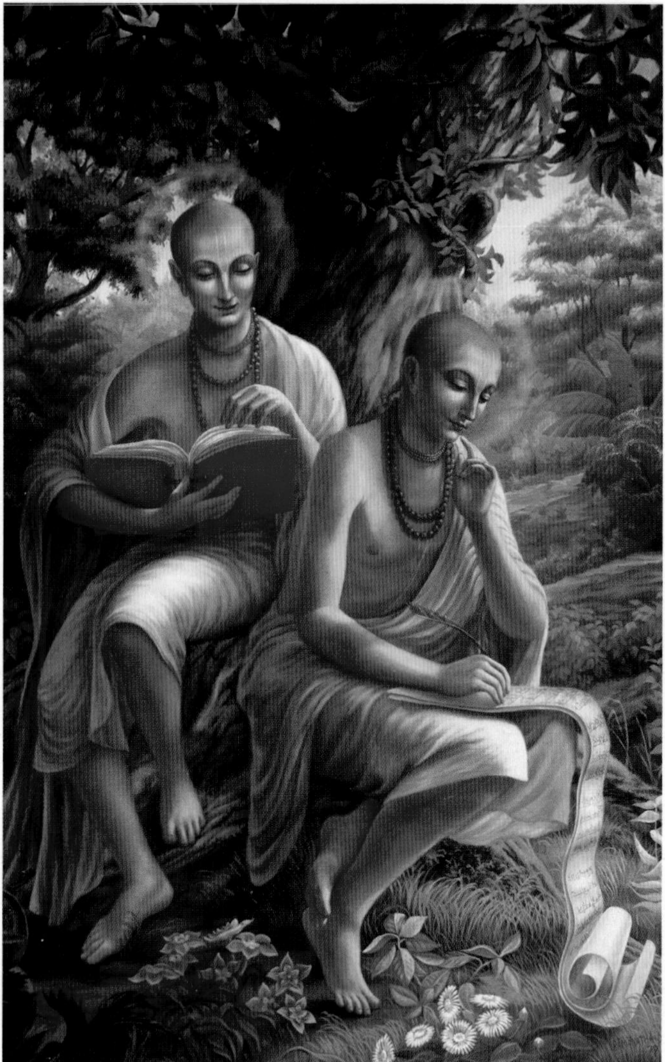

Śrīla Rūpa Gosvāmī (*right*), the author of the *Bhakti-rasāmṛta-sindhu*, and Śrīla Sanātana Gosvāmi (*left*), his elder brother and spiritual master—leaders of the Six Gosvāmīs of Vṛndāvana (p. 1)

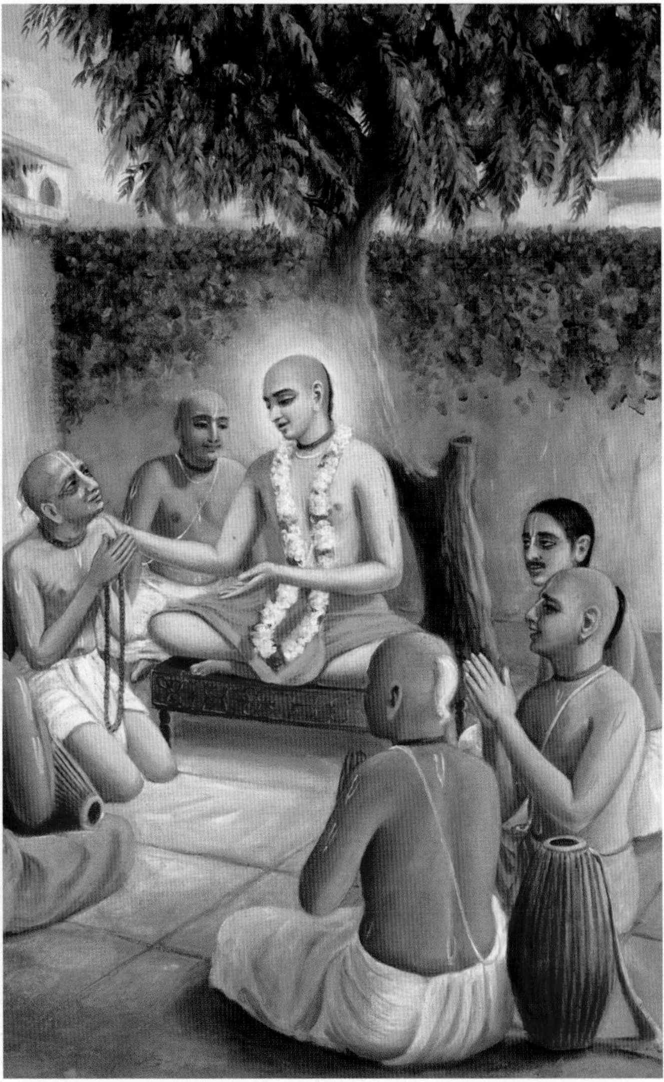

Lord Caitanya, who is Kṛṣṇa, the Supreme Personality of Godhead, playing the part of His own devotee, instructed His followers on the science of Kṛṣṇa consciousness. (p. 2)

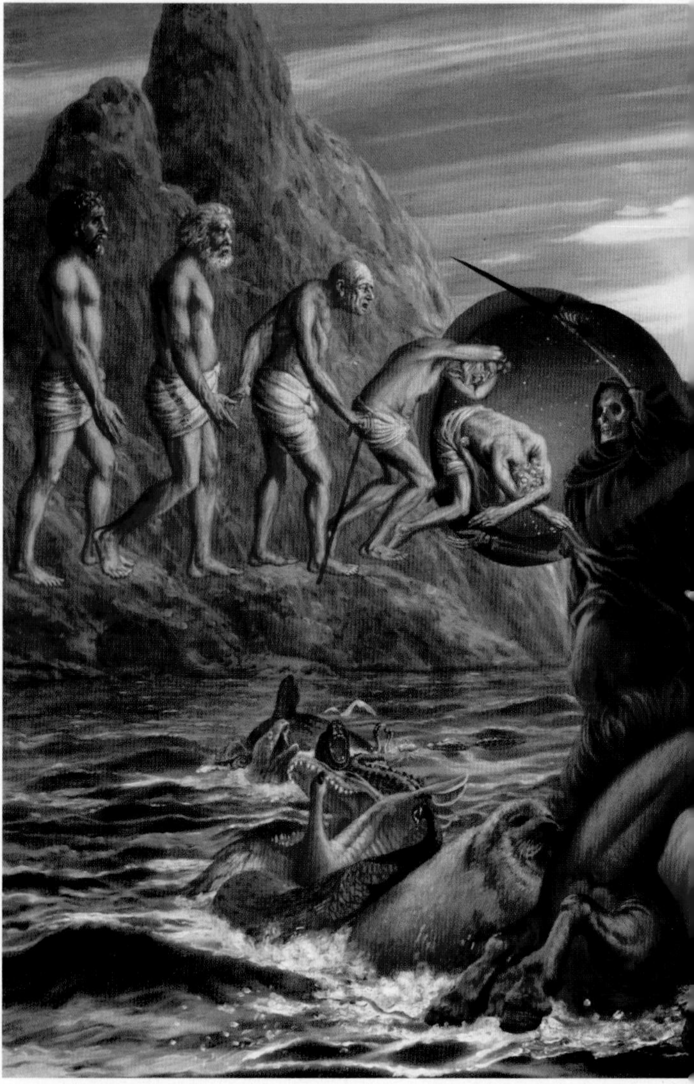

"*Daiva* supervision gives us a body selected from 8,400,000 forms; the choice does not depend on our selection, but is awarded to us according to our destiny." (p. 5)

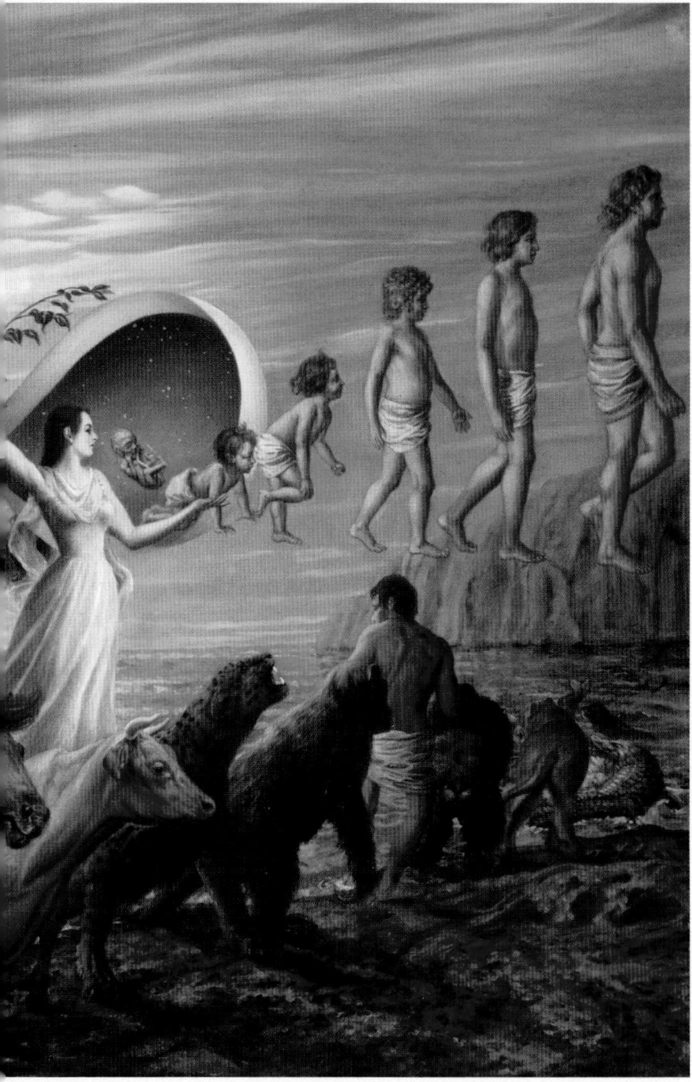

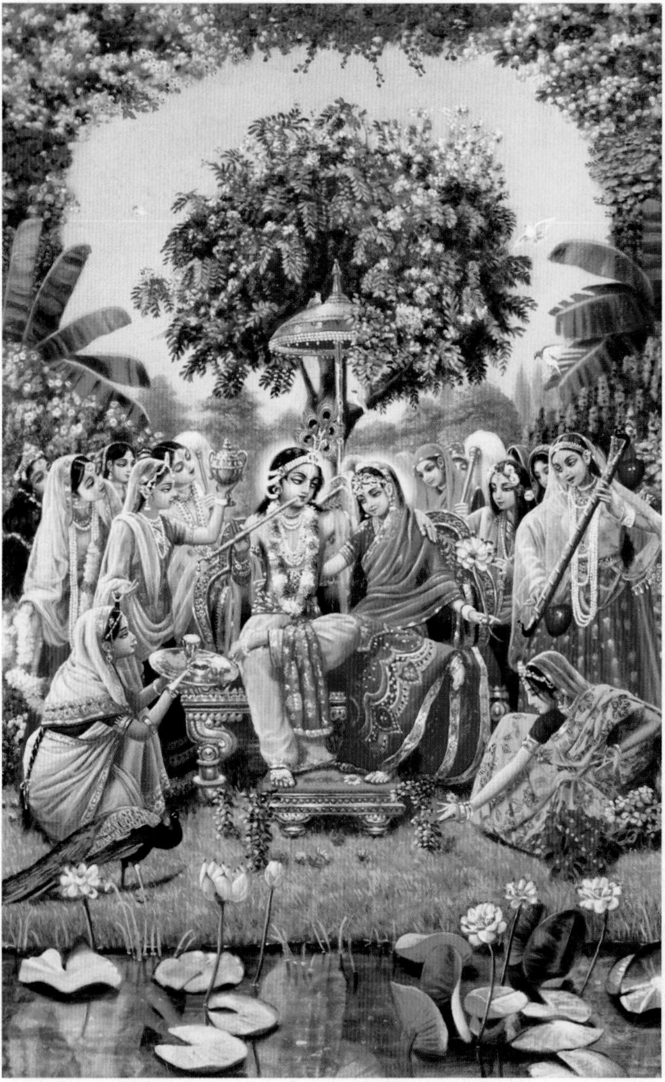

We all have a propensity to love someone. *Bhakti-yoga* teaches us how to reawaken our love for Kṛṣṇa and enjoy blissful spiritual life. (p. 6)

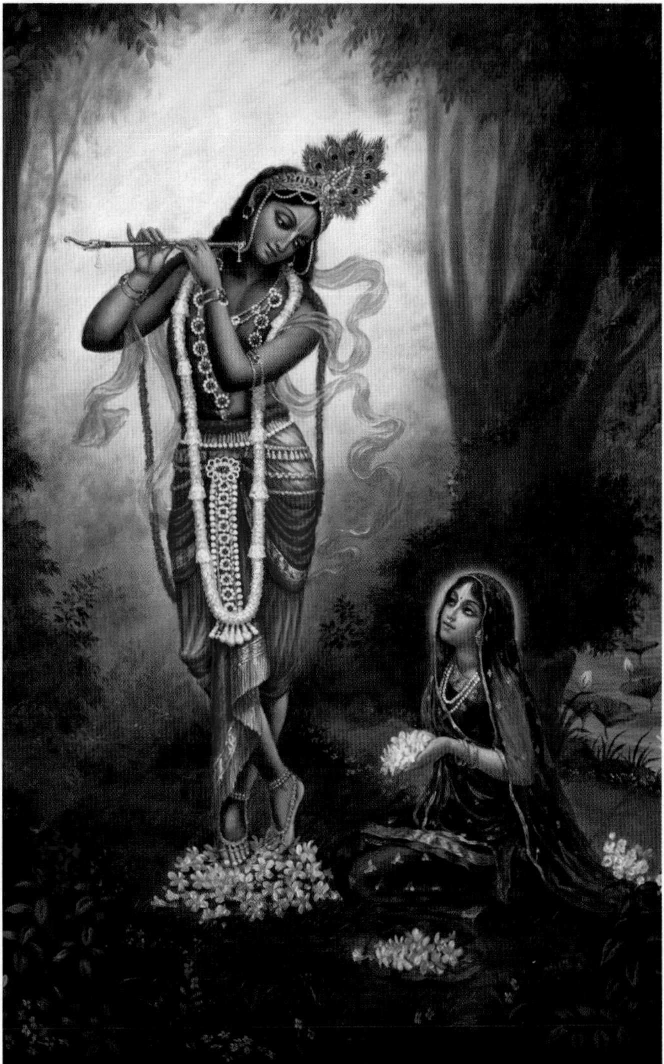

Śrīmatī Rādhārāṇī, Lord Kṛṣṇa's eternal consort, is the queen of *bhakti*. (p. 30)

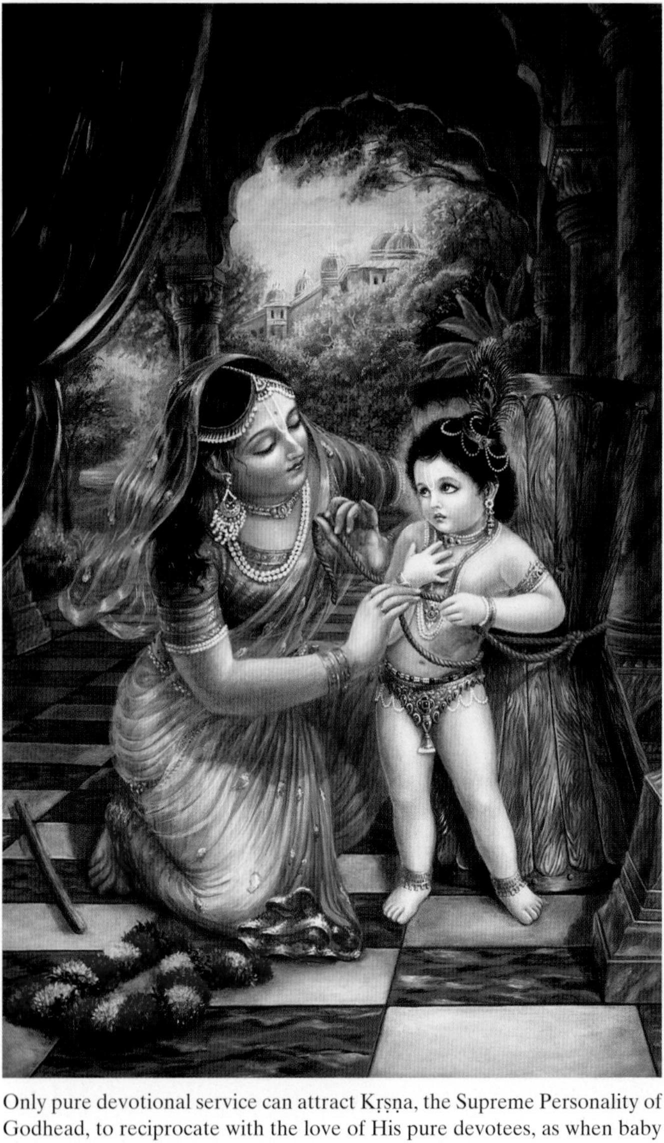

Only pure devotional service can attract Kṛṣṇa, the Supreme Personality of Godhead, to reciprocate with the love of His pure devotees, as when baby Kṛṣṇa allowed Himself to be bound by his mother, Yaśodā. (p. 32)

A Pure Devotee Wants Nothing But Bhakti

In the *Hari-bhakti-sudhodaya* it is stated that Prahlāda Mahārāja, a great devotee of the Lord, prayed to Nṛsiṁhadeva (the half-lion, half-man incarnation) as follows: "My dear Lord, I repeatedly pray unto Your lotus feet that I may simply be stronger in devotional service. I simply pray that my Kṛṣṇa consciousness may be more strong and steady, because happiness derived from Kṛṣṇa consciousness and devotional service is so powerful that with it one can have all the other perfections of religiousness, economic development, sense gratification, and even the attainment of liberation from material existence."

Actually, a pure devotee does not aspire after any of these perfections, because the happiness derived from devotional service in Kṛṣṇa consciousness is so transcendental and so unlimited that no other happiness can compare to it. It is said that even one drop of happiness in Kṛṣṇa consciousness stands beyond comparison with an ocean of happiness derived from any other activity. Thus, any person who has developed even a little quantity of pure devotional service can very easily kick out all the other kinds of happiness derived from religiousness, economic development, sense gratification, and liberation.

There was a great devotee of Lord Caitanya known as Kholāvecā Śrīdhara, who was a very poor man. He was doing a small business selling cups made from the leaves of plantain trees, and his income was almost nothing. Still, he was spending fifty percent of his small income on the worship of the Ganges, and with the other fifty percent he was somehow living. Lord Caitanya once revealed Himself to this confidential devotee, Kholāvecā Śrīdhara, and offered him any opulence he liked. But Śrīdhara informed the Lord that he did not want any material opulence. He was quite happy in his present position and wanted only to gain unflinching faith and devotion unto the lotus feet of Lord Caitanya. That is the position of pure devotees. If they can be engaged twenty-four hours each day in devotional service, they do not want anything else, not even the happiness of liberation or of becoming one with the Supreme.

In the *Nārada-pañcarātra* it is also said that any person who has developed even a small amount of devotional service doesn't care a fig for any kind of happiness derived from religiousness, economic development, sense gratification, or the five kinds of liberation. Any kind of happiness derived from religiousness, economic development, liberation, or sense gratification cannot even dare to enter into the heart of a pure devotee. It is stated that as the personal attendants and maidservants of a queen follow the queen with all respect and obeisances, similarly the joys of religiousness, economic development, sense gratification, and liberation follow the devotional service of the Lord. In other words, a pure devotee does not lack any kind of happiness derived from any source. He does not want anything but service to Kṛṣṇa, but even if he should have another desire, the Lord fulfills it without the devotee's asking.

(4)
The Rarity of Pure Devotional Service

In the preliminary phase of spiritual life there are different kinds of austerities, penances, and similar processes for attaining self-realization. However, even if an executor of these processes is without any material desire, he still cannot achieve devotional service. And aspiring by oneself alone to achieve devotional service is also not very hopeful, because Kṛṣṇa does not agree to award devotional service to merely anyone. Kṛṣṇa can easily offer a person material happiness or even liberation, but He does not agree very easily to award a person engagement in His devotional service. Devotional service can in fact be attained only through the mercy of a pure devotee. In the *Caitanya-caritāmṛta* (*Madhya* 19.151) it is said, "By the mercy of the spiritual master who is a pure devotee and by the mercy of Kṛṣṇa one can achieve the platform of devotional service. There is no other way."

The rarity of devotional service is also confirmed in the *tantra-śāstra,* where Lord Śiva says to Satī, "My dear Satī, if one is a very fine philosopher, analyzing the different processes of knowledge, he can achieve liberation from material entanglement. By performance of the ritualistic sacrifices recommended in the *Vedas* one can be elevated to the platform of pious activities and thereby enjoy the material comforts of life to the fullest extent. But all such endeavors can hardly offer anyone devotional service to the Lord, not even if one tries for it by such processes for many, many thousands of births."

In the *Śrīmad-Bhāgavatam* Prahlāda Mahārāja confirms that merely by personal efforts or by the instructions of higher authorities one cannot attain to the stage of devotional service. One must become blessed by the dust of the lotus feet of a pure devotee, who is completely freed from the contamination of material desires.

Tasting the Honey of Bhakti

Devotional service is dependent on the mercy of Kṛṣṇa and His devotees. Unless we surrender to the lotus feet of a pure devotee, it is not possible to come to the platform of pure devotional service. By his own efforts a bee cannot taste the honey within a bottle. The bottle must be opened by a superior. If the bee simply licks the outside of the bottle, thinking, "Now I am tasting honey," then he is in illusion. Similarly, no one can enter into devotional service unless the door is opened by a devotee. Therefore Rūpa Gosvāmī says, *ādau gurvāśrayam:* The first step in devotional service is to accept a guru from a disciplic succession that follows the principles of *bhakti*. Then you will very easily enter onto the path of devotional service. You have to select a guru who is *niṣkiñcana,* "free of material desires." One who has accepted the lotus feet of the Lord has finished with all material desires. Such a pure devotee wants only to be engaged in the Lord's service in whatever condition of life he is in.

King Yudhiṣṭhira was such a pure devotee. In the Fifth Canto of *Śrīmad-Bhāgavatam* (5.6.18) Nārada says to Yudhiṣṭhira, "My dear king, it is Lord Kṛṣṇa, known as Mukunda, who is the eternal protector of the Pāṇḍavas and the Yadus. He is also your spiritual master and instructor in every respect. He is the only worshipable God for you. He is very dear and affectionate, and He is the director of all your activities, both individual and familial. And what's more, He sometimes carries out your orders as if He were your messenger! My dear king, how very fortunate you are, because for others all these favors given to you by the Supreme Lord would not even be dreamt of." The purport to this verse is that the Lord easily offers liberation but He rarely agrees to offer a soul devotional service, because by devotional service the Lord Himself becomes purchased by the devotee.

(5)
Bhakti Minimizes the Happiness of Becoming One with the Supreme

Śrīla Rūpa Gosvāmī says that if *brahmānanda,* or the happiness of becoming one with the Supreme, is multiplied by one trillionfold, it still cannot compare to an atomic fraction of the happiness derived from the ocean of devotional service.

In the *Hari-bhakti-sudhodaya* Prahlāda Mahārāja, while satisfying Lord Nṛsiṁhadeva with his prayers, says, "My dear Lord of the universe, I am feeling transcendental pleasure in Your presence and have become merged in the ocean of happiness. I now consider the happiness of *brahmānanda* to be no more than the water in the impression left by a cow's hoof in the earth, compared to this ocean of bliss." Similarly, it is confirmed in the *Bhāvārtha-dīpikā,* Śrīdhara Svāmī's commentary on the *Śrīmad-Bhāgavatam,* "My dear Lord, some of the fortunate persons who are swimming in the ocean of Your nectar of devotion, and who are relishing the nectar of the narration of Your pastimes, certainly know ecstasies that immediately minimize the value of the happiness derived from religiousness, economic development, sense gratification, and liberation. Such a transcendental devotee regards any kind of happiness other than devotional service as no better than straw in the street."

(6)
Only Bhakti Can Attract Kṛṣṇa

Śrīla Rūpa Gosvāmī has stated that devotional service attracts even Kṛṣṇa. Kṛṣṇa attracts everyone, but devotional service attracts Kṛṣṇa. The symbol of devotional service in the highest degree is Rādhārāṇī. Kṛṣṇa is called Madana-mohana, which means that He is so attractive that He can defeat the attraction of thousands of Cupids. But Rādhārāṇī is still more attractive, for She can attract even Kṛṣṇa. Therefore devotees call Her Madana-mohana-mohinī—the attractor of the attractor of Cupid.

Madana means sex attraction. So since Kṛṣṇa is Madana-mohana, one can neglect even sex attraction if one is attracted to Kṛṣṇa. Sex attracts everyone in this material world. Indeed, the whole material world is running on sex, and so-called happiness begins from sexual intercourse. Generally, a man marries to satisfy his sex desire. In that way, he begets children. When the children are grown, they marry and have more children. It is all for the same purpose: sex. Material happiness means these three things: *śrī* (a beautiful woman), *aiśvarya* (wealth), and *prajā* (offspring). Generally, people want a good wife, a good bank balance, and a good family. If a man has these things, he is considered successful.

Through the effort to acquire and maintain a wife, children, friends, and wealth, the attraction for this material world becomes tighter and tighter. We should avoid being attracted by the glitter of this material world and try to become attracted by Kṛṣṇa. In this connection, Śrī Yāmunācārya said,

yad-avadhi mama cetaḥ kṛṣṇa-pādāravinde
nava-nava-rasa-dhāmany udyataṁ rantum āsīt
tad-avadhi bata nārī-saṅgame smaryamāne
bhavati mukha-vikāraḥ suṣṭhu niṣṭhīvanaṁ ca

"Since I have been attracted by the beauty of Kṛṣṇa and have begun to serve His lotus feet, I am experiencing an ever-new taste. Therefore, as soon as I think of sexual intercourse, my lips curl with distaste and I want to spit." When one is attracted by Kṛṣṇa, Cupid is defeated and one conquers over this material world. Otherwise, the material world is very difficult to surpass. But if anyone grabs Kṛṣṇa's lotus feet very strongly, calling out, "Kṛṣṇa, save me!" Kṛṣṇa promises, "I will save you. Do not worry." In the *Bhagavad-gītā* Kṛṣṇa tells Arjuna, "You can declare to the world, I will protect My pure devotee." People do not know that their only business is to take shelter of the lotus feet of Kṛṣṇa and thus achieve the aim of human life, which is to get out of the clutches of the material world. Any other business means we are becoming entangled in this material world.

Śrīmatī Rādhārāṇī, the Queen of Bhakti

To perform devotional service means to follow in the footsteps of Rādhārāṇī, and devotees in Vṛndāvana put themselves under the care of Rādhārāṇī in order to achieve perfection in their devotional service. In other words, devotional service is not an activity of the material world; it is directly under the control of Rādhārāṇī. In the *Bhagavad-gītā* it is confirmed that the *mahātmās,* or great souls, are under the protection of *daivī prakṛti,* the internal energy—Rādhārāṇī. So, being directly under the control of the internal potency of Kṛṣṇa, devotional service attracts even Kṛṣṇa Himself.

This fact is corroborated by Kṛṣṇa in the Eleventh Canto of *Śrīmad-Bhāgavatam* (11.14.20), where He says, "My dear Uddhava, you may know it from Me that the attraction I feel for devotional service rendered by My devotees is not to be attained even by the performance of mystic yoga, philosophical speculation, ritualistic sacrifices, the study of *Vedānta,* the practice of severe austerities, or the giving of everything in charity. These are, of course, very nice activities, but they are not as attractive to Me as the transcendental loving service rendered by My devotees."

How Kṛṣṇa becomes attracted by the devotional service of His devotees is described by Nārada Muni in the Seventh Canto of *Śrīmad-Bhāgavatam* (7.10.48–49). There Nārada addresses King Yudhiṣṭhira while the king is appreciating the glories of the character of Prahlāda Mahārāja. A devotee always appreciates the activities of other devotees. Yudhiṣṭhira Mahārāja was appreciating the qualities of Prahlāda, and that appreciation is one symptom of a pure devotee. A pure devotee never thinks himself great; he always thinks that other devotees are greater than himself. The king was thinking, "Prahlāda Mahārāja is actually a devotee of the Lord, while I am nothing," and while thinking this he was addressed by Nārada as follows: "My dear King Yudhiṣṭhira, you [the Pāṇḍava brothers] are the only fortunate people in this world. The Supreme Personality of Godhead has appeared on this planet and is presenting Himself to you as an ordinary human being. He is always with you in all circumstances. He is living with you and covering Himself from the eyes of others. Others cannot understand that He is the Supreme Lord, but He is still living with you as your cousin, as your friend, and even as your messenger. Therefore you must know that nobody in this world is more fortunate than you."

In the *Bhagavad-gītā,* when Kṛṣṇa appeared in His universal form Arjuna prayed, "My dear Kṛṣṇa, I thought of You as my cousin-brother, and so I have shown disrespect to You in so many ways, calling You 'Kṛṣṇa' or 'friend.' But You are so great that I could not understand." So that was the position of the Pāṇḍavas: although Kṛṣṇa is the Supreme Personality of Godhead, the greatest among all greats, He remained with those royal brothers, being attracted by their devotion, by their friendship, and by their love. That is the proof of how great this process of devotional service is. It can attract even the Supreme Personality of Godhead. God is great, but devotional service is greater than God because it attracts Him. People who are not in devotional service can never understand what great value there is in rendering service to the Lord.

Bhakti-yoga at Home

by Mahātmā Dāsa

In *Bhakti-yoga, the Art of Eternal Love,* Śrīla Prabhupāda makes it clear how important it is for everyone to practice *bhakti-yoga,* devotional service to Lord Kṛṣṇa. Of course, living in the association of Kṛṣṇa's devotees in a temple or ashram makes it easier to practice devotional service. But if you're determined, you can follow at home the teachings of *bhakti-yoga,* or Kṛṣṇa consciousness, and thus convert your home into a temple.

Spiritual life, like material life, means practical activity. The difference is that whereas we perform material activities for the benefit of ourselves or those we consider ours, we perform spiritual activities for the benefit of Lord Kṛṣṇa, under the guidance of the scriptures and the spiritual master. The key is to accept the guidance of the scripture and the guru. Kṛṣṇa declares in the *Bhagavad-gītā* that a person can achieve neither happiness nor the supreme destination of life—going back to Godhead, back to Lord Kṛṣṇa—if he or she does not follow the injunctions of the scriptures. And *how* to follow the scriptural rules by engaging in practical service to the Lord—that is explained by a bona fide spiritual master. Without following the instructions of a spiritual master who is in an authorized chain of disciplic succession coming from Kṛṣṇa Himself, we cannot make spiritual progress. The practices outlined here are the timeless practices of *bhakti-yoga* as given by the foremost spiritual master and exponent of Kṛṣṇa consciousness in our time, His Divine Grace A. C. Bhaktivedanta Swami Prabhupāda, founder-*ācārya* of the International Society for Krishna Consciousness (ISKCON).

The purpose of spiritual knowledge is to bring us closer to God, or Kṛṣṇa. Kṛṣṇa says in the *Bhagavad-gītā* (18.55), *bhaktyā māṁ abhijānāti:* "I can be known only by devotional service." Knowledge guides us in proper action. Spiritual knowledge directs us to satisfy the desires of Kṛṣṇa through practical engagements in His loving service. Without practical application, theoretical knowledge is of little value.

Spiritual knowledge is meant to direct us in all aspects of life. We should endeavor, therefore, to organize our lives in such a way as to follow Kṛṣṇa's teachings as far as possible. We should try to do our best, to do more than is simply convenient. Then it will be possible for us to rise to the transcendental plane of Kṛṣṇa consciousness, even while living far from a temple.

Chanting the Hare Kṛṣṇa Mantra

The first principle in devotional service is to chant the Hare Kṛṣṇa *mahā-mantra* (*mahā* means "great"; *mantra* means "sound that liberates the mind from ignorance"):

> Hare Kṛṣṇa, Hare Kṛṣṇa, Kṛṣṇa Kṛṣṇa, Hare Hare
> Hare Rāma, Hare Rāma, Rāma Rāma, Hare Hare

You should chant these holy names of the Lord as much as possible—anywhere and at any time—but it is also very helpful to set a specific time of the day to regularly chant. Early morning hours are ideal.

The chanting can be done in two ways: singing the mantra, called *kīrtana* (usually done in a group), and saying the mantra to oneself, called *japa* (which literally means "to speak softly"). Concentrate on hearing the sound of the holy names. As you chant, pronounce the names clearly and distinctly, addressing Kṛṣṇa in a prayerful mood. When your mind wanders, bring it back to the sound of the Lord's names. Chanting is a prayer to Kṛṣṇa that means "O energy of the Lord [Hare], O all-attractive Lord [Kṛṣṇa], O Supreme Enjoyer [Rāma], please engage me in Your service." The more attentively and sincerely you chant these names of God, the more spiritual progress you will make. Since God is all-powerful and all-merciful, He has kindly made it very easy for us to chant His names, and He has also invested all His powers in them. Therefore the names of God and God Himself are identical. This means that when we chant the holy names of Kṛṣṇa and Rāma we are directly associating with God and being purified. Therefore we should always try to chant with devotion and reverence. The Vedic literature states that Lord Kṛṣṇa is personally dancing on your tongue when you chant His holy name.

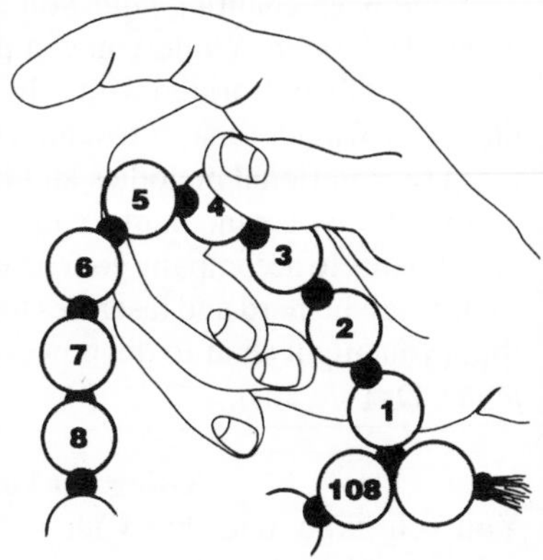

When you chant alone, it is best to chant on *japa* beads (call the mailorder branch of the Bhaktivedanta Book Trust, at 1-800-927-4152). This not only helps you fix your attention on the holy name, but it also helps you count the number of times you chant the mantra daily. Each strand of *japa* beads contains 108 small beads and one large bead, the head bead. Begin on a bead next to the head bead and gently roll it between the thumb and middle finger of your right hand as you chant the full Hare Kṛṣṇa mantra. Then move to the next bead and repeat the process. In this way, chant on each of the 108 beads until you reach the head bead again. This is one round of *japa*. Then, without chanting on the head bead, reverse the beads and start your second round on the last bead you chanted on.

Initiated devotees vow before the spiritual master to chant at least sixteen rounds of the Hare Kṛṣṇa mantra daily. But even if you can chant only one round a day, the principle is that once you commit yourself to chanting that round, you should try to complete it every day without fail. When you feel you can chant more, then increase the minimum number of rounds you chant each day—but don't fall below that number. You can chant more than your fixed number, but you should maintain a set minimum each day. (Please note that the beads are sacred and therefore should never touch the ground or be put in an unclean place. To keep your beads clean, it's best to carry them in a special bead bag, such as the one that comes as part of the Mantra Meditation Kit.)

Aside from chanting *japa,* you can also sing the Lord's holy names in *kīrtana.* While you can perform *kīrtana* individually, it is generally performed with others. A melodious *kīrtana* with family or friends is sure to enliven everyone. ISKCON devotees use traditional melodies and instruments, especially in the temple, but you can chant to any melody and use any musical instruments to accompany your chanting. As Lord Caitanya said, "There are no hard and fast rules for chanting Hare Kṛṣṇa." One thing you might want to do, however, is order some *kīrtana* and *japa* CDs (see ads).

Setting Up Your Altar

You will likely find that your *japa* and *kīrtana* are especially effective when done before an altar. Lord Kṛṣṇa and His pure devotees are so kind that they allow us to worship them even through their pictures. It is something like mailing a letter: You cannot mail a letter by placing it in just any box; you must use the mailbox authorized by the government. Similarly, we cannot imagine a picture of God and worship that, but we can worship the authorized picture of God, and Kṛṣṇa accepts our worship through that picture.

Setting up an altar at home means receiving the Lord and His pure devotees as your most honored guests. Where should you set up the altar? Well, how would you seat a guest? An ideal place would be clean, well lit, and free from drafts and household disturbances. Your guest, of course, would need a comfortable chair, but for the picture of Kṛṣṇa's form a wall shelf, a mantelpiece, a corner table, or the top shelf of a bookcase will do. You wouldn't seat a guest in your home and then ignore him; you'd provide a place for yourself to sit, too, where you could comfortably face him and enjoy his company. So don't make your altar inaccessible.

What do you need for an altar? Here are the essentials:

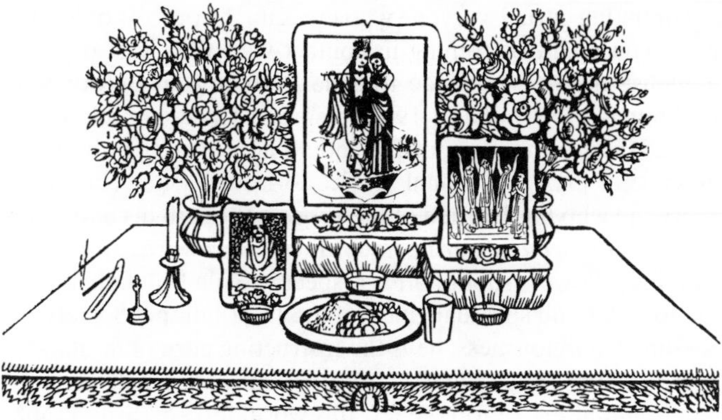

1. A picture of Śrīla Prabhupāda.
2. A picture of Lord Caitanya and His associates.
3. A picture of Śrī Śrī Rādhā-Kṛṣṇa.

In addition, you may want an altar cloth, water cups (one for each picture), candles with holders, a special plate for offering food, a small bell, incense, an incense holder, and fresh flowers, which you may offer in vases or simply place beforeeach picture. If you're interested in more elaborate Deity worship, ask any of the ISKCON devotees or get in touch with the BBT (call 1-800-927-4152 or visit www.krishna.com).

The first person we worship on the altar is the spiritual master. The spiritual master is not God. Only God is God. But because the spiritual master is His dearmost servant, God has empowered him, and therefore he deserves the same respect as that given to God. He links the disciple with God and teaches him the process of *bhakti-yoga.* He is God's ambassador to the material world. When a president sends an ambassador to a foreign country, the ambassador receives the same respect as that accorded the president, and the ambassador's words are as authoritative as the president's. Similarly, we should respect the spiritual master as we would God, and revere his words as we would His.

There are two main kinds of gurus: the instructing guru and

the initiating guru. Everyone who takes up the process of *bhakti-yoga* as a result of coming in contact with ISKCON owes an immense debt of gratitude to Śrīla Prabhupāda. Before Śrīla Prabhupāda left India in 1965 to spread Kṛṣṇa consciousness abroad, almost no one outside India knew anything about the practice of pure devotional service to Lord Kṛṣṇa. Therefore, everyone who has learned of the process through his books, his *Back to Godhead* magazine, recordings of his words, or contact with his followers should offer respect to Śrīla Prabhupāda. As the founder and spiritual guide of the International Society for Krishna Consciousness, he is the instructing guru of us all.

As you progress in *bhakti-yoga,* you may eventually want to accept initiation. Before he left this world in 1977, Śrīla Prabhupāda encouraged his qualified disciples to carry on his work by initiating disciples of their own in accordance with his instructions. At present there are many spiritual masters in ISKCON. To learn how you can get spiritual guidance from them, ask a devotee at your nearby temple, or write to one of the ISKCON centers listed at the end of this book.

The second picture on your altar should be one of the *pañca-tattva,* Lord Caitanya and His four leading associates. Lord Caitanya is the incarnation of God for this age. He is Kṛṣṇa Himself, descended in the form of His own devotee to teach us how to surrender to Him, specifically by chanting His holy names and performing other activities of *bhakti-yoga.* Lord Caitanya is the most merciful incarnation, for He makes it easy for anyone to attain love of God through the chanting of the Hare Kṛṣṇa *mantra*.

And of course your altar should have a picture of the Supreme Personality of Godhead, Lord Śrī Kṛṣṇa, with His eternal consort, Śrīmatī Rādhārāṇī. Śrīmatī Rādhārāṇī is Kṛṣṇa's spiritual potency. She is devotional service personified, and devotees always take shelter of Her to learn how to serve Kṛṣṇa.

You can arrange the pictures in a triangle, with the picture of Śrīla Prabhupāda on the left, the picture of Lord Caitanya and

His associates on the right, and the picture of Rādhā and Kṛṣṇa, which, if possible, should be slightly larger than the others, on a small raised platform behind and in the center. Or you can hang the picture of Rādhā and Kṛṣṇa on the wall above.

Carefully clean the altar each morning. Cleanliness is essential in Deity worship. Remember, you wouldn't neglect to clean the room of an important guest, and when you establish an altar you invite Kṛṣṇa and His pure devotees to reside as the most exalted guests in your home. If you have water cups, rinse them out and fill them with fresh water daily. Then place them conveniently close to the pictures. You should remove flowers in vases as soon as they're slightly wilted, or daily if you've offered them at the base of the pictures. You should offer fresh incense at least once a day, and, if possible, light candles and place them near the pictures when you're chanting before the altar.

Please try the things we've suggested so far. It's very simple, really: If you try to love God, you'll gradually realize how much He loves you. That's the essence of *bhakti-yoga.*

Prasādam: How to Eat Spiritually

By His immense transcendental energies, Kṛṣṇa can actually convert matter into spirit. If we place an iron rod in a fire, before long the rod becomes red hot and acts just like fire. In the same way, food prepared for and offered to Kṛṣṇa with love and devotion becomes completely spiritualized. Such food is called Kṛṣṇa *prasādam,* which means "the mercy of Lord Kṛṣṇa."

Eating *prasādam* is a fundamental practice of *bhakti-yoga.* In other forms of yoga one must artificially repress the senses, but the *bhakti-yogī* can engage his or her senses in a variety of pleasing spiritual activities, such as tasting delicious food offered to Lord Kṛṣṇa. In this way the senses gradually become spiritualized and bring the devotee more and more transcendental pleasure by being engaged in devotional service. Such spiritual pleasure far surpasses any material experience.

Lord Caitanya said of *prasādam,* "Everyone has tasted these foods before. However, now that they have been prepared for Kṛṣṇa and offered to Him with devotion, these foods have acquired extraordinary tastes and uncommon fragrances. Just taste them and see the difference in the experience! Apart from the taste, even the fragrance pleases the mind and makes one forget any other fragrance. Therefore, it should be understood that the spiritual nectar of Kṛṣṇa's lips must have touched these ordinary foods and imparted to them all their transcendental qualities."

Eating only food offered to Kṛṣṇa is the perfection of vegetarianism. In itself, being a vegetarian is not enough; after all, even pigeons and monkeys are vegetarians. But when we go beyond vegetarianism to a diet of *prasādam,* our eating becomes helpful in achieving the goal of human life—reawakening the soul's original relationship with God. In the *Bhagavad-gītā* Lord Kṛṣṇa says that unless one eats only food that has been offered to him in sacrifice, one will suffer the reactions of karma.

How to Prepare and Offer Prasādam

As you walk down the supermarket aisles selecting the foods you will offer to Kṛṣṇa, you need to know what is offerable and what is not. In the *Bhagavad-gītā,* Lord Kṛṣṇa states, "If one offers Me with love and devotion a leaf, a flower, a fruit, or water, I will accept it." From this verse it is understood that we can offer Kṛṣṇa foods prepared from milk products, vegetables, fruits, nuts, and grains. (Call 1-800-927-4152 or check out krishna.com for Hare Kṛṣṇa cookbooks.) Meat, fish, and eggs are not offerable. And a few vegetarian items are also forbidden—garlic and onions, for example, which are in the mode of darkness. (Hing, or asafetida, is a tasty substitute for them in cooking and is available at most Indian groceries and ISKCON temple stores.) Nor can you offer to Kṛṣṇa coffee or tea that contain caffeine. If you like these beverages, purchase caffeine-free coffee and herbal teas.

While shopping, be aware that you may find meat, fish, and egg products mixed with other foods; so be sure to read labels carefully. For instance, some brands of yogurt and sour cream contain gelatin, a substance made from the horns, hooves, and bones of slaughtered animals. Also, make sure the cheese you buy contains no animal rennet, an enzyme from the stomach tissues of slaughtered calves. Most hard cheese sold in America contains this rennet, so be careful about any cheese you can't verify as being free from animal rennet.

Also avoid foods cooked by nondevotees. According to the subtle laws of nature, the cook acts upon the food not only physically but mentally as well. Food thus becomes an agent for subtle influences on your consciousness. The principle is the same as that at work with a painting: a painting is not simply a collection of strokes on a canvas but an expression of the artist's state of mind, which affects the viewer. So if you eat food cooked by nondevotees—employees working in a factory, for example—then you're sure to absorb a dose of materialism and karma. So as far as possible use only fresh, natural ingredients.

In preparing food, cleanliness is the most important principle. Nothing impure should be offered to God; so keep your kitchen very clean. Always wash your hands thoroughly before entering the kitchen. While preparing food, do not taste it, for you are cooking the meal not for yourself but for the pleasure of Kṛṣṇa. Arrange portions of the food on dinnerware kept especially for this purpose; no one but the Lord should eat from these dishes. The easiest way to offer food is simply to pray, "My dear Lord Kṛṣṇa, please accept this food," and to chant each of the following prayers three times while ringing a bell (see the Sanskrit Pronunciation Guide on page 62):

1. Prayer to Śrīla Prabhupāda:

nama oṁ viṣṇu-pādāya kṛṣṇa-preṣṭhāya bhū-tale
śrīmate bhaktivedānta- svāminn iti nāmine

namas te sārasvate deve gaura-vāṇī-pracāriṇe
nirviśeṣa-śūnyavādi- pāścātya-deśa-tāriṇe

"I offer my respectful obeisances unto His Divine Grace A. C. Bhaktivedanta Swami Prabhupāda, who is very dear to Lord Kṛṣṇa on this earth, having taken shelter at His lotus feet. Our respectful obeisances are unto you, O spiritual master, servant of Bhaktisiddhānta Sarasvatī Gosvāmī. You are kindly preaching the message of Lord Caitanyadeva and delivering the Western countries, which are filled with impersonalism and voidism."

2. Prayer to Lord Caitanya:

namo mahā-vadānyāya kṛṣṇa-prema-pradāya te
kṛṣṇāya kṛṣṇa-caitanya- nāmne gaura-tviṣe namaḥ

"O most munificent incarnation! You are Kṛṣṇa Himself appearing as Śrī Kṛṣṇa Caitanya Mahāprabhu. You have assumed the golden color of Śrīmatī Rādhārāṇī, and You are widely distributing pure love of Kṛṣṇa. We offer our respectful obeisances unto You."

3. Prayer to Lord Kṛṣṇa:

namo brahmaṇya-devāya go-brāhmaṇa-hitāya ca
jagad-dhitāya kṛṣṇāya govindāya namo namaḥ

"I offer my respectful obeisances unto Lord Kṛṣṇa, who is the worshipable Deity for all *brāhmaṇas,* the well-wisher of the cows and the *brāhmaṇas,* and the benefactor of the whole world. I offer my repeated obeisances to the Personality of Godhead, known as Kṛṣṇa and Govinda."

Remember that the real purpose of preparing and offering food to the Lord is to show your devotion and gratitude to Him. Kṛṣṇa accepts your devotion, not the physical offering itself. God is complete in Himself—He doesn't need anything—but out of His immense kindness He allows us to offer food to Him so that we can develop our love for Him.

After offering the food to the Lord, wait at least five minutes for Him to partake of the preparations. Then you should transfer the food from the special dinnerware and wash the dishes and utensils you used for the offering. Now you and any guests may eat the *prasādam*. While you eat, try to appreciate the spiritual value of the food. Remember that because Kṛṣṇa has accepted it, it is nondifferent from Him, and therefore by eating it you will become purified.

Everything you offer on your altar becomes *prasādam,* the mercy of the Lord. Flowers, incense, the water, the food—everything you offer for the Lord's pleasure becomes spiritualized. The Lord enters into the offerings, and thus the remnants are nondifferent from Him. So you should not only deeply respect the things you've offered, but you should distribute them to others as well. Distribution of *prasādam* is an essential part of Deity worship.

Everyday Life: The Four Regulative Principles

Anyone serious about progressing in Kṛṣṇa consciousness must try to avoid the following four sinful activities:

1. Eating meat, fish, or eggs. These foods are saturated with the modes of passion and ignorance and therefore cannot be offered to the Lord. A person who eats these foods participates in a conspiracy of violence against helpless animals and thus stops his spiritual progress dead in its tracks.

2. Gambling. Gambling invariably puts one into anxiety and fuels greed, envy, and anger.

3. The use of intoxicants. Drugs, alcohol, and tobacco, as well as any drinks or foods containing caffeine, cloud the mind, overstimulate the senses, and make it impossible to xunderstand or follow the principles of *bhakti-yoga*.

4. Illicit sex. This is sex outside of marriage or sex in marriage for any purpose other than procreation. Sex for pleasure

compels one to identify with the body and takes one far from Kṛṣṇa consciousness. The scriptures teach that sex is the most powerful force binding us to the material world. Anyone serious about advancing in Kṛṣṇa consciousness should minimize sex or eliminate it entirely.

Engagement in Practical Devotional Service

Everyone must do some kind of work, but if you work only for yourself you must accept the karmic reactions of that work. As Lord Kṛṣṇa says in the *Bhagavad-gītā* (3.9), "Work done as a sacrifice for Viṣṇu [Kṛṣṇa] has to be performed. Otherwise work binds one to the material world."

You needn't change your occupation, except if you're now engaged in a sinful job such as working as a butcher or bartender. If you're a writer, write for Kṛṣṇa; if you're an artist, create for Kṛṣṇa; if you're a secretary, type for Kṛṣṇa. You may also directly help the temple in your spare time, and you should sacrifice some of the fruits of your work by contributing a portion of your earnings to help maintain the temple and propagate Kṛṣṇa consciousness. Some devotees living outside the temple buy Hare Kṛṣṇa literature and distribute it to their friends and associates, or they engage in a variety of services at the temple. There is also a wide network of devotees who gather in each other's homes for chanting, worship, and study. Write to your local temple or the Society's secretary to learn of any such programs near you.

Additional Devotional Principles

There are many more devotional practices that can help you become Kṛṣṇa conscious. Here are two vital ones:

Studying Hare Kṛṣṇa Literature

Śrīla Prabhupāda, the founder-*ācārya* of ISKCON, dedicated much of his time to writing books such as the *Bhagavad-gītā As It Is* and *Śrīmad-Bhāgavatam,* both of which are quoted extensively in *Spiritual Yoga*. Hearing the words—or reading the writings—

of a realized spiritual master is an essential spiritual practice. So try to set aside some time every day to read Śrīla Prabhupāda's books. You can get a free catalog of available books and other media from the BBT.

Associating with Devotees

Śrīla Prabhupāda established the Hare Kṛṣṇa movement to give people in general the chance to associate with devotees of the Lord. This is the best way to gain faith in the process of Kṛṣṇa consciousness and become enthusiastic in devotional service. Conversely, maintaining intimate connections with nondevotees slows one's spiritual progress. So try to visit the Hare Kṛṣṇa center nearest you as often as possible.

In Closing

The beauty of Kṛṣṇa consciousness is that you can take as much as you're ready for. Kṛṣṇa Himself promises in the *Bhagavad-gītā* (2.40), "There is no loss or diminution in this endeavor, and even a little advancement on this path protects one from the most fearful type of danger." So bring Kṛṣṇa into your daily life, and we guarantee you'll feel the benefit.

Hare Kṛṣṇa!

SANSKRIT PRONUNCIATION GUIDE

The system of transliteration used in this book conforms to a system that scholars have accepted to indicate the pronunciation of each sound in the Sanskrit language.

The short vowel **a** is pronounced like the **u** in b**u**t, long **ā** like the **a** in f**a**r. Short **i** is pronounced as in p**i**n, long **ī** as in p**i**que, short **u** as in p**u**ll, and long **ū** as in r**u**le. The vowel **ṛ** is pronounced like the **ri** in **ri**m, **e** like the **ey** in th**ey**, **o** like the **o** in g**o**, **ai** like the **ai** in **ai**sle, and **au** like the **ow** in h**ow**. The *anusvāra* (**ṁ**) is pronounced like the **n** in the French word *bo***n**, and *visarga* (**ḥ**) is pronounced as a final **h** sound. At the end of a couplet, **aḥ** is pronounced **aha**, and **iḥ** is pronounced **ihi**.

The guttural consonants—**k, kh, g, gh,** and **ṅ**—are pronounced from the throat in much the same manner as in English. **K** is pronounced as in **k**ite, **kh** as in Ec**kh**art, **g** as in **g**ive, **gh** as in di**g h**ard, and **ṅ** as in si**ng.**

The palatal consonants—**c, ch, j, jh,** and **ñ**—are pronounced with the tongue touching the firm ridge behind the teeth. **C** is pronounced as in **ch**air, **ch** as in staun**ch-h**eart, **j** as in **j**oy, **jh** as in he**dgeh**og, and **ñ** as in ca**ny**on.

The cerebral consonants—**ṭ, ṭh, ḍ, ḍh,** and **ṇ**—are pronounced with the tip of the tongue turned up and drawn back against the dome of the palate. **Ṭ** is pronounced as in **t**ub, **ṭh** as in ligh**t-h**eart, **ḍ** as in **d**ove, **ḍh** as in re**d-h**ot, and **ṇ** as in **n**ut. The dental consonants—**t, th, d, dh,** and **n**—are pronounced in the same manner as the cerebrals, but with the forepart of the tongue against the teeth.

The labial consonants—**p, ph, b, bh,** and **m**—are pronounced with the lips. **P** is pronounced as in **p**ine, **ph** as in u**ph**ill, **b** as in **b**ird, **bh** as in ru**b-h**ard, and **m** as in **m**other.

The semivowels—**y, r, l,** and **v**—are pronounced as in **y**es, **r**un, **l**ight, and **v**ine respectively. The sibilants—**ś, ṣ,** and **s**—are pronounced, respectively, as in the German word *sprechen* and the English words **sh**ine and **s**un. The letter **h** is pronounced as in **h**ome.

Glossary

Ācārya—an ideal teacher who knows the revealed scriptures, behaves exactly according to their injunctions, and teaches his students to adopt these principles also.

Arjuna—an eternal associate of Kṛṣṇa.

Bhagavad-gītā—a seven-hundred-verse record of a conversation between Lord Kṛṣṇa and His disciple Arjuna, recorded in the *Mahābhārata*.

Bhakti-rasāmṛta-sindhu—one of the principal works on the science of *bhakti-yoga,* written by Śrīla Rūpa Gosvāmī in the sixteenth century.

Bhakti-yoga—the system of cultivation of *bhakti,* or pure devotional service to God, which is untinged by sense gratification or philosophical speculation.

Brāhmaṇa—a member of the intellectual, priestly class; a person wise in Vedic knowledge, fixed in goodness, and knowledgeable of Brahman, the Absolute Truth.

Caitanya-caritāmṛta—the foremost biography of Lord Caitanya Mahāprabhu. Written in Bengali and Sanskrit in the late sixteenth century by Śrīla Kṛṣṇadāsa Kavirāja Gosvāmī, it brilliantly presents the Lord's pastimes and teachings.

Caitanya Mahāprabhu (1486–1534)—Lord Kṛṣṇa in the aspect of His own devotee. He appeared in Navadvīpa, West Bengal, and inaugurated the congregational chanting of the holy names of the Lord to teach pure love of God.

Disciplic succession—a chain of spiritual masters and their disciples who in turn became spiritual masters.

False ego—the conception that "I am this material body, mind, or intelligence."

Gosvāmī—a person who has his senses under full control.

Guru—spiritual master.

Haridāsa Ṭhākura—a confidential associate of Śrī Caitanya Mahāprabhu who, though born in a Muslim family, was so absorbed in the nectar of chanting the holy name of Kṛṣṇa that he chanted day and night.

Kurukṣetra—a place of pilgrimage about ninety miles north of New Delhi where Lord Kṛṣṇa spoke the *Bhagavad-gītā* to Arjuna five thousand years ago. It was here that the great *Mahābhārata* war was fought.

Liberation—freedom from birth and death.

Mahā-mantra—"the great mantra": Hare Kṛṣṇa, Hare Kṛṣṇa, Kṛṣṇa Kṛṣṇa, Hare Hare/ Hare Rāma, Hare Rāma, Rāma Rāma, Hare Hare.

Māyāvādī—an impersonalist.

Nārada Muni—a pure devotee of the Lord, one of the sons of Lord Brahmā, who travels throughout the universes in his eternal body, glorifying devotional service while delivering the science of *bhakti*. He is the spiritual master of Vyāsadeva and of many other great devotees.

Nārada-pañcarātra—Nārada Muni's book on the processes of Deity worship and mantra meditation.

Pāṇḍavas—the five pious *kṣatriya* brothers Yudhiṣṭhira, Bhīma, Arjuna, Nakula, and Sahadeva. They were intimate friends of Lord Kṛṣṇa's and inherited the leadership of the world upon their victory over the Kurus in the Battle of Kurukṣetra.

Prahlāda Mahārāja—a great devotee of Lord Kṛṣṇa who was persecuted by his demonic father Hiraṇyakaśipu but was protected by the Lord and ultimately saved by Him in the form of Nṛsiṁhadeva, the Lord's half-man, half-lion incarnation.

Rādhārāṇī—Lord Kṛṣṇa's most intimate consort, who personifies His pleasure potency.

Rūpa Gosvāmī—chief of the Six Gosvāmīs of Vṛndāvana, who were empowered by Lord Caitanya to establish the philosophy of Kṛṣṇa consciousness.

Sanātana Gosvāmī—one of the Six Gosvāmīs of Vṛndāvana, who were empowered by Lord Caitanya to establish the philosophy of Kṛṣṇa consciousness. He was the older brother of Rūpa Gosvāmī, who accepted him as his spiritual master.

Satī—the wife of Lord Śiva and the daughter of Dakṣa. She burned herself alive when her father insulted her husband.

Self-realization—the understanding that one is not the body but a spirit soul and that one is an eternal servant of Kṛṣṇa.

Śiva, Lord—the demigod who supervises the material mode of ignorance (*tamo-guṇa*) and who annihilates the material cosmos.

Six Gosvāmīs—six renounced followers of Śrī Caitanya Mahāprabhu whom He deputed to go to Vṛndāvana to excavate the places of Kṛṣṇa's pastimes and write books on Kṛṣṇa consciousness.

Śrīmad-Bhāgavatam—the foremost of the eighteen *Purāṇas.* The complete science of God, it establishes the supreme position of Lord Kṛṣṇa.

Supreme Brahman—the Personality of Godhead, Lord Śrī Kṛṣṇa.

Tantra-śāstra—Vedic literatures consisting mostly of dialogues between Lord Śiva and Durgā. They contain instructions on Deity worship and other aspects of spiritual practice.

Vedānta—the philosophy of the *Vedānta-sūtra* of Śrīla Vyāsadeva, containing a conclusive summary of Vedic philosophical knowledge and showing Kṛṣṇa as the goal.

Vedas—the four original scriptures (*Ṛg, Sāma, Atharva,* and *Yajur*).

Vṛndāvana—Kṛṣṇa's eternal abode, where He fully manifests His quality of sweetness; the village on this earth where He enacted His childhood pastimes five thousand years ago.

Yadus—the descendants of Yadu. They constitute the dynasty in which Lord Kṛṣṇa appeared.

Yāmunācārya—a great Vaiṣṇava spiritual master and author in the Śrī-sampradāya, one of the important disciplic lines of Vaiṣṇavas.

Yoga, mystic—meditative yoga.

Yudhiṣṭhira—the eldest of the Pāṇḍavas in the *Mahābhārata,* and the son of Dharmarāja or Yamarāja, the god of death.

The International Society for Krishna Consciousness
Founder-Ācārya: His Divine Grace A.C. Bhaktivedanta Swami Prabhupāda

CENTERS AROUND THE WORLD

(Partial List)

CANADA

Brampton-Mississauga, Ontario — Unit 20, 1030 Kamato Dr., L4W 4B6/Tel. (416) 840-6587 or (905) 826-1290/ iskconbrampton@gmail.com

Calgary, Alberta — 313 Fourth St. N.E., T2E 3S3/ Tel. (403) 265-3302/ Fax: (403) 547-0795/vamanstones@shaw.ca

Edmonton, Alberta — 9353 35th Ave. NW, T6E 5R5/ Tel. (780) 439-9999/ harekrishna.edmonton@gmail.com

Montreal, Quebec — 1626 Pie IX Blvd., H1V 2C5/ Tel. & fax: (514) 521-1301/ iskconmontreal@gmail.com

♦ **Ottawa, Ontario** — 212 Somerset St. E., K1N 6V4/ Tel. (613) 565-6544/ Fax: (613) 565-2575/iskconottawa@sympatico.ca

Regina, Saskatchewan — 1279 Retallack St., S4T 2H8/ Tel. (306) 525-0002 or -6461/jagadishadas@yahoo.com

Toronto, Ontario — 243 Avenue Rd., M5R 2J6/ Tel. (416) 922-5415/ Fax: (416) 922-1021/ toronto@iskcon.net

Vancouver, B.C. — 5462 S.E. Marine Dr., Burnaby V5J 3G8/ Tel. (604) 433-9728/ Fax: (604) 648-8715/akrura@krishna.com; Govinda's Bookstore & Cafe/ Tel. (604) 433-7100 or 1-888-433-8722

RURAL COMMUNITY

Ashcroft, B.C. — Saranagati Dhama, Venables Valley (mail: P.O. Box 99, V0K 1A0)/ Tel. (250) 457-7438/Fax: (250) 453-9306/ iskconsaranagati@hotmail.com

U.S.A.

Atlanta, Georgia — 1287 South Ponce de Leon Ave. N.E., 30306/ Tel. & fax: (404) 377-8680/ admin@atlantaharekrishnas.com

Austin, Texas — 10700 Jonwood Way, 78753/ Tel. (512) 835-2121/ Fax: (512) 835-8479/ sda@backtohome.com

Baltimore, Maryland —200 Bloomsbury Ave., Catonsville, 21228/ Tel. (410) 719-1776/ Fax: (410) 799-0642/ info@baltimorekrishna.com

Berkeley, California — 2334 Stuart St., 94705/ Tel. (510) 649-8619/ Fax: (510) 665-9366/ rajan416@yahoo.com

Boise, Idaho — 1615 Martha St., 83706/ Tel. (208) 344-4274/ boise_temple@yahoo.com

Boston, Massachusetts — 72 Commonwealth Ave., 02116/ Tel. (617) 247-8611/ Fax: (617) 909-5181/ darukrishna@iskconboston.org

Chicago, Illinois — 1716 W. Lunt Ave., 60626/ Tel. (773) 973-0900/ Fax: (773) 973-0526/ chicagoiskcon@yahoo.com

Columbus, Ohio — 379 W. Eighth Ave., 43201/ Tel. (614) 421-1661/ Fax: (614) 294-0545/ rmanjari@sbcglobal.net

♦ **Dallas, Texas** — 5430 Gurley Ave., 75223/ Tel. (214) 827-6330/ Fax: (214) 823-7264/ txkrishnas@aol.com; restaurant: vegetariantaste@aol.com

♦ **Denver, Colorado** — 1400 Cherry St., 80220/ Tel. (303) 333-5461/ Fax: (303) 321-9052/ info@krishnadenver.com

Detroit, Michigan — 383 Lenox Ave., 48215/ Tel. (313) 824-6000/ gaurangi108@hotmail.com

Gainesville, Florida — 214 N.W. 14th St., 32603/ Tel. (352) 336-4183/ Fax: (352) 379-2927/ kalakantha.acbsp@pamho.net

Hartford, Connecticut — 1683 Main St., E. Hartford 06108/ Tel. & fax: (860) 289-7252/ pyari@sbcglobal.net

♦ **Honolulu, Hawaii** — 51 Coelho Way, 96817/ Tel. (808) 595-4913/ rama108@bigfoot.com

Houston, Texas — 1320 W. 34th St., 77018/ Tel. (713) 686-4482/ Fax: (713) 956-9968/ management@iskconhouston.org

Kansas City, Missouri — 5201 Paseo Blvd./ Tel. (816) 924-5619/ Fax: (816) 924-5640/ rvc@rvc.edu

Laguna Beach, California — 285 Legion St., 92651/ Tel. (949) 494-7029/ info@lagunatemple.com

Las Vegas, Nevada — Govinda's Center of Vedic India, 6380 S. Eastern Ave., Suite 8, 89120/ Tel. (702) 434-8332/ info@govindascenter.com

♦ **Los Angeles, California** — 3764 Watseka Ave., 90034/ Tel. (310) 836-2676/ Fax: (310) 839-2715/ membership@harekrishnala.com

♦ **Miami, Florida** — 3220 Virginia St., 33133 (mail: 3109 Grand Ave. #491, Coconut Grove, FL 33133)/ Tel. (305) 442-7218/ devotionalservice@iskcon-miami.org

New Orleans, Louisiana — 2936 Esplanade Ave., 70119/ Tel. (504) 304-0032 (office) or (504) 638-3244/ iskcon.new.orleans@pamho.net

♦ **New York, New York** — 305 Schermerhorn St., Brooklyn 11217/ Tel. (718) 855-6714/ Fax: (718) 875-6127/ ramabhadra@aol.com

New York, New York — 26 Second Ave., 10003/ Tel. (212) 253-6182/ krishnanyc@gmail.com

Orlando, Florida — 2651 Rouse Rd., 32817/ Tel. (407) 257-3865

Philadelphia, Pennsylvania — 41 West Allens Lane, 19119/ Tel. (215) 247-4600/ Fax: (215) 247-8702/ savecows@aol.com

♦ **Philadelphia, Pennsylvania** — 1408 South St., 19146/ Tel. (215) 985-9303/ savecows@aol.com

Phoenix, Arizona — 100 S. Weber Dr., Chandler, 85226/ Tel. (480) 705-4900/ Fax: (480) 705-4901/ svgd108@yahoo.com

Portland, Oregon — 2095 NW Alocleck Dr., Suites 1107 & 1109, Hillsboro 97124/ Tel. (503) 439-9117/ info@iskconportland.com

St. Augustine, Florida — 3001 First St., 32084/ Tel. & fax: (904) 819-0221/ vasudeva108@gmail.com

♦ **St. Louis, Missouri** — 3926 Lindell Blvd., 63108/ Tel. (314) 535-8085 or 534-1708/ Fax: (314) 535-0672/ rpsdas@gmail.com

San Antonio, Texas — 6772 Oxford Trace, 78240/ Tel. (210) 401-6576/ aadasa@gmail.com

♦ **San Diego, California** — 1030 Grand Ave., Pacific Beach 92109/ Tel. (310) 895-0104/ Fax: (858) 483-0941/ krishna.sandiego@gmail.com

San Jose, California — 951 S. Bascom Ave., 95128/ Tel. (408) 293-4959/ iskconsanjose@yahoo.com

Seattle, Washington — 1420 228th Ave. S.E., Sammamish 98075/ Tel. (425) 246-8436/ Fax: (425) 868-8928/ info@vedicculturalcenter.org

♦ **Spanish Fork, Utah** — Krishna Temple Project & KHQN Radio, 8628 S. State Rd., 84660/ Tel. (801) 798-3559/ Fax: (810) 798-9121/ carudas@earthlink.net

Tallahassee, Florida — 1323 Nylic St., 32304/ Tel. & fax: (850) 224-3803/ darudb@hotmail.com

Towaco, New Jersey — 100 Jacksonville Rd. (mail: P.O. Box 109), 07082/ Tel. & fax: (973) 299-0970/ newjersey@iskcon.net

♦ **Tucson, Arizona** — 711 E. Blacklidge Dr., 85719/ Tel. (520) 792-0630/ Fax: (520) 791-0906/ tucphx@cs.com

Washington, D.C. — 10310 Oaklyn Dr., Potomac, Maryland 20854/ Tel. (301) 299-2100/ Fax: (301) 299-5025/ ad@pamho.net

RURAL COMMUNITIES

♦ **Alachua, Florida (New Raman Reti)** — 17306 N.W. 112th Blvd., 32615 (mail: P.O. Box 819, 32616)/ Tel. (386) 462-2017/ Fax: (386) 462-2641/ alachuatemple@gmail.com

Carriere, Mississippi (New Talavan) — 31492 Anner Road, 39426/ Tel. (601) 749-9460 or 799-1354/ Fax: (601) 799-2924/ talavan@hughes.net

Gurabo, Puerto Rico (New Govardhana Hill) — Carr. 181, Km. 16.3, Bo. Santa Rita, Gurabo (mail: HC-01, Box 8440, Gurabo,

♦ Temples with restaurants or dining

PR 00778)/ Tel. (787) 367-3530 or (787) 737-1722/ manonath@gmail.com

Hillsborough, North Carolina (New Goloka) — 1032 Dimmocks Mill Rd., 27278/ Tel. (919) 732-6492/ bkgoswami@earthlink.net

Moundsville, West Virginia (New Vrindaban) — R.D. No. 1, Box 319, Hare Krishna Ridge, 26041/ Tel. (304) 843-1600; Visitors, (304) 845-5905/ Fax: (304) 845-0023/ mail@newvrindaban.com

Mulberry, Tennessee (Murari-sevaka) — 532 Murari Lane, 37359 (mail: P.O. Box 108, Lynchburg, TN 37352)/ Tel. (931) 227-6156/ Tel. & fax: (931) 759-6888/ murari_sevaka@yahoo.com

Port Royal, Pennsylvania (Gita Nagari) — 534 Gita Nagari Rd./ Tel. (717) 527-4101/ kaulinidasi@hotmail.com

Sandy Ridge, North Carolina — Prabhupada Village, 1283 Prabhupada Rd., 27046/ Tel. (336) 593-9888/ madanmohanmohinni@yahoo.com

ADDITIONAL RESTAURANTS

Hato Rey, Puerto Rico — Tamal Krishna's Veggie Garden, 131 Eleanor Roosevelt, 00918/ Tel. (787) 754-6959/ Fax: (787) 756-7769/ tkveggiegarden@aol.com

Seattle, Washington — My Sweet Lord, 5521 University Way, 98105/ Tel. (425) 643-4664

UNITED KINGDOM AND IRELAND

Belfast, Northern Ireland — Brooklands, 140 Upper Dunmurray Lane, BT17 OHE/ Tel. +44 (28) 9062 0530

Birmingham, England — 84 Stanmore Rd., Edgbaston B16 9TB/ Tel. +44 (121) 420 4999/ birmingham@iskcon.org.uk

Cardiff, Wales — The Soul Centre, 116 Cowbridge Rd., East Canton CF11 9DX/ Tel. +44 (29) 2039 0391/ the.soul.centre@pamho.net

Coventry, England — Kingfield Rd., Coventry (mail: 19 Gloucester St., Coventry CV1 3BZ)/ Tel. +44 (24) 7655 2822 or 5420/ haridas.kds@pamho.net

• **Dublin, Ireland** — 83 Middle Abbey St., Dublin 1/ Tel. +353 (1) 661 5095/ dublin@krishna.ie; Govinda's: info@govindas.ie

Lesmahagow, Scotland — Karuna Bhavan, Bankhouse Rd., Lesmahagow, Lanarkshire, ML11 0ES/ Tel. +44 (1555) 894790/ Fax: +44 (1555) 894526/ karunabhavan@aol.com

Leicester, England — 21 Thoresby St., North Evington, LE5 4GU/ Tel. +44 (116) 276 2587/ pradyumna.jas@pamho.net

• **London, England (city)** — 10 Soho St., W1D 3DL/ Tel. +44 (20) 7437-3662; residential /pujaris, 7439-3606; shop, 7287-0269; Govinda's Restaurant, 7437-4928/ Fax: +44 (20) 7439-1127/ london@pamho.net

• **London, England (country)** — Bhaktivedanta Manor, Dharam Marg, Hilfield Lane, Watford, Herts, WD25 8EZ/ Tel. +44 (1923) 851000/ Fax: +44 (1923) 851006/ info@krishnatemple.com; Guesthouse: bmguesthouse@krishna.com

London, England (south) — 42 Enmore Road, South Norwood, SE25 5NG/ Tel. +44 7988857530/ krishnaprema89@hotmail.com

London, England (Kings Cross) — 102 Caledonain Rd., Kings Cross, Islington, N1 9DN/ Tel. +44 (20) 7168 5732/ foodforalluk@aol.com

Manchester, England — 20 Mayfield Rd., Whalley Range, M16 8FT/ Tel. +44 (161) 226 4416/ contact@iskconmanchester.com

Newcastle-upon-Tyne, England — 304 Westgate Rd., NE4 6AR/ Tel. +44 (191) 272 1911

• **Swansea, Wales** — 8 Craddock St., SA1 3EN/ Tel. +44 (1792) 468469/ iskcon.swansea@pamho.net (restaurant: govindas@hotmail.com)

RURAL COMMUNITIES

Upper Lough Erne, Northern Ireland — Govindadwipa Dhama, Inisrath Island, Derrylin, Co. Fermanagh, BT92 9GN/ Tel. +44 (28) 6772 1512/ govindadwipa@pamho.net

London, England — (contact Bhaktivedanta Manor) Programs are held regularly in more than forty other cities in the UK. For information, contact ISKCON Reader Services, P.O. Box 730, Watford WD25 8EZ, UK; www.iskcon.org.uk

ADDITIONAL RESTAURANTS

Dublin, Ireland — Govinda's, 4 Aungier St., Dublin 2/ Tel. +353 (1) 475 0309/ Fax: +353 (1) 478 6204/ info@govindas.ie

Dublin, Ireland — Govinda's, 18 Merrion Row, Dublin 2/ Tel. +353 (1) 661 5095/ praghosa.sdg@pamho.net

AUSTRALASIA

AUSTRALIA

Adelaide — 25 Le Hunte St. (mail: P.O. Box 114, Kilburn, SA 5084)/ Tel. & fax: +61 (8) 8359-5120/ iskconsa@tpg.com.au

Brisbane — 95 Bank Rd., Graceville (mail: P.O. Box 83, Indooroopilly), QLD 4068/ Tel. +61 (7) 3379-5455/ Fax: +61 (7) 3379-5880/ brisbane@iskcon.org.au

Canberra — 1 Quick St., Ainslie, ACT 2602 (mail: P.O. Box 1411, Canberra, ACT 2601)/ Tel. & fax: +61 (2) 6262-6208/ iskcon@harekrishnacanberra.com

Melbourne — 197 Danks St. (mail: P.O. Box 125), Albert Park, VIC 3206/ Tel. +61 (3) 9699-5122/ Fax: +61 (3) 9690-4093/ melbourne@pamho.net

Newcastle — 28 Bull St., Mayfield, NSW 2304/ Tel. +61 (2) 4967-7000/ iskcon_newcastle@yahoo.com.au

Perth — 155–159 Canning Rd., Kalamunda (mail: P.O. Box 201 Kalamunda 6076)/ Tel. +61 (8) 6293-1519/ perth@pamho.net

Sydney — 180 Falcon St., North Sydney, NSW 2060 (mail: P.O. Box 459, Cammeray, NSW 2062)/ Tel. +61 (2) 9959-4558/ Fax: +61 (2) 9957-1893/ admin@iskcon.com.au

Sydney — Govinda's Yoga & Meditation Centre, 112 Darlinghurst Rd., Darlinghurst NSW 2010 (mail: P.O. Box 174, Kings Cross 1340)/ Tel. +61 (2) 9380-5162/ Fax: +61 (2) 9360-1736/ sita@govindas.com.au

RURAL COMMUNITIES

Bambra, VIC (New Nandagram) — 50 Seaches Outlet, off 1265 Winchelsea Deans Marsh Rd., Bambra VIC 3241/ Tel. +61 (3) 5288-7383

Cessnock, NSW (New Gokula) — Lewis Lane (Off Mount View Road, Millfield, near Cessnock [mail: P.O. Box 399, Cessnock, NSW 2325])/ Tel. +61 (2) 4998-1800/ Fax: (Sydney temple)/ iskconfarm@mac.com

Murwillumbah, NSW (New Govardhana) — Tyalgum Rd., Eungella (mail: P.O. Box 687), NSW 2484/ Tel. +61 (2) 6672-6579/ Fax: +61 (2) 6672-5498/ ajita@in.com.au

RESTAURANTS

Brisbane — Govinda's, 99 Elizabeth St., 1st Floor, QLD 4000/ Tel. +61 (7) 3210-0255

Brisbane — Krishna's Cafe, 1st Floor, 82 Vulture St., W. End, QLD 4000/ brisbane@pamho.net

Burleigh Heads — Govindas, 20 James St., Burleigh Heads, QLD 4220/ Tel. +61 (7) 5607-0782/ ajita@in.com.au

Cairns — Gaura Nitai's, 55 Spence St., Cairns, QLD/ Tel. +61 (7) 4031-2255 or (425) 725 901/ Fax: +61 (7) 4031 2256/ gauranitais@in.com.au

Maroochydore — Govinda's Vegetarian Cafe, 2/7 First Ave., QLD 4558/ Tel. +61 (7) 5451-0299

Melbourne — Crossways, 1st Floor, 123 Swanston St., VIC 3000/ Tel. +61 (3) 9650-2939

Melbourne — Gopal's, 139 Swanston St., VIC 3000/ Tel. +61 (3) 9650-1578

Newcastle — Govinda's Vegetarian Cafe, 110 King St., corner of

King & Wolf Streets, NSW 2300/ Tel. +61 (2) 4929-6900 / info@govindascafe.com.au

Perth — Hare Krishna Food for Life, 200 William St., Northbridge, WA 6003/ Tel. +61 (8) 9227-1684/ iskconperth@optusnet.com.au

NEW ZEALAND AND FIJI

Auckland, NZ — The Loft, 1st Floor, 103 Beach Rd./ Tel. +64 (9) 3797301

Christchurch, NZ — 83 Bealey Ave. (mail: P.O. Box 25-190)/ Tel. +64 (3) 366-5174/ Fax: +64 (3) 366-1965/ iskconchch@clear.net.nz

Hamilton, NZ — 188 Maui St., RD 8, Te Rapa/ Tel. +64 (7) 850-5108/ rmaster@wave.co.nz

Labasa, Fiji — Delailabasa (mail: P.O. Box 133)/ Tel. +679 812912

Lautoka, Fiji — 5 Tavewa Ave. (mail: P.O. Box 125)/ Tel. +679 666 4112/ regprakash@excite.com

Nausori, Fiji — Hare Krishna Cultural Centre, 2nd Floor, Shop & Save Building 11 Gulam Nadi St., Nausori Town (mail: P.O. Box 2183, Govt. Bldgs., Suva)/ Tel. +679 9969748 or 3475097/ Fax: +679 3477436/ vdas@frca.org.fj

Rakiraki, Fiji — Rewasa (mail: P.O. Box 204)/ Tel. +679 694243

Sigatoka, Fiji — Queens Rd., Olosara (mail: P.O. Box 1020)/ Tel. +679 6520866 or 6500349/ drgsmarna@connect.com.fj

Suva, Fiji — 166 Brewster St. (mail: P.O. Box 4229, Samabula)/ Tel. +679 331 8441/ Fax: +679 3100016/ iskconsuva@connect.com.fj

Wellington, NZ — 105 Newlands Rd., Newlands/ Tel. +64 (4) 478-4108/ info@iskconwellington.org.nz

Wellington, NZ — Gaura Yoga Centre, 1st Floor, 175 Vivian St. (mail: P.O. Box 6271, Marion Square)/ Tel. +64 (4) 801-5500/ yoga@gaurayoga.co.nz

RURAL COMMUNITY

Auckland, NZ (New Varshan) — Hwy. 28, Riverhead, next to Huapai Golf Course (mail: R.D. 2, Kumeu)/ Tel. +64 (9) 412-8075/ Fax: +64 (9) 412-7130

RESTAURANTS

Auckland, NZ — Hare Krishna Food for Life, 268 Karangahape Rd./ Tel. +64 (9) 300-7585

Labasa, Fiji — Hare Krishna Restaurant, Naseakula Road/ Tel. +679 811364

Lautoka, Fiji — Gopal's, Corner of Yasawa Street and Naviti Street/ Tel. +679 662990

Suva, Fiji — Hare Krishna Vegetarian Restaurant, Dolphins FNPF Place, Victoria Parade/ Tel. +679 314154/ vdas@govnet.gov.fj

Suva, Fiji — Hare Krishna Vegetarian Restaurant, Opposite University of the South Pacific, Laucala Bay Rd./ Tel. +679 311683/ vdas@govnet.gov.fj

Suva, Fiji — Hare Krishna Vegetarian Restaurant, 18 Pratt St./ Tel. +679 314154

Suva, Fiji — Hare Krishna Vegetarian Restaurant, 82 Ratu Mara Rd., Samabula/ Tel. +679 386333

Suva, Fiji — Hare Krishna Vegetarian Restaurant, Terry Walk, Cumming St./ Tel. +679 312295

Wellington, NZ — Higher Taste Hare Krishna Restaurant, Old Bank Arcade, Ground Flr., Corner Customhouse, Quay & Hunter St., Wellington/ Tel. +64 (4) 472-2233/ Fax: (4) 472-2234/ highertaste@iskconwellington.orgorg.nz

INDIA (partial list)*

Ahmedabad, Gujarat — Satellite Rd., Gandhinagar Highway Crossing, 380 054/ Tel. (079) 686-1945, -1645, or -2350/ jasomatinandan.acbsp@pamho.net

Allahabad, UP — Hare Krishna Dham, 161 Kashi Raj Nagar, Baluaghat 211 003/ Tel. (0532) 415294

Amritsar, Punjab — Chowk Moni Bazar, Laxmansar, 143 001/ Tel. (0183) 2540177

Bangalore, Karnataka — Hare Krishna Hill, Chord Rd., 560 010/ Tel. (080) 23471956 or 23578346/ Fax: (080) 23578625/ manjunath36@iskconbangalore.org

Bangalore, Karnataka — ISKCON Sri Jagannath Mandir, No.5 Sripuram, 1st cross, Sheshadripuram, Bangalore 560 020/ Tel. (080) 3536867 or 2262024 or 3530102

Baroda, Gujarat — Hare Krishna Land, Gotri Rd., 390 021/ Tel. (0265) 2310630 or 2331012/ iskcon.baroda@pamho.net

• **Bhubaneswar, Orissa** — N.H. No. 5, IRC Village, 751 015/ Tel. (0674) 2553517, 2553475, or 2554283

Chandigarh, Punjab — Hare Krishna Dham, Sector 36-B, 160 036/ Tel. (0172) 601590 or 603232/ iskcon.chandigarh@pamho.net

Chennai (Madras), TN — Hare Krishna Land, Bhaktivedanta Swami Road, Off ECR Road, Injam- bakkam, Chennai 600 041/ Tel. (044) 5019303 or 5019147/ iskconchennai@eth.net

• **Coimbatore, TN** — Jagannath Mandir, Hare Krishna Land, Aerodrome P.O., Opp. CIT, 641 014/ Tel. (0422) 2626509 or 2626508/ info@iskcon-coimbatore.org

Dwarka, Gujarat — Bharatiya Bhavan, Devi Bhavan Rd., 361 335/ Tel. (02892) 34606/ Fax: (02892) 34319

Guwahati, Assam — Ulubari Chariali, South Sarania, 781 007/ Tel. (0361) 2525963/ iskcon.guwahati@pamho.net

Haridwar, Uttaranchal — Prabhupada Ashram, G. House, Nai Basti, Mahadev Nagar, Bhimgoda/ Tel. (01334) 260818

Hyderabad, AP — Hare Krishna Land, Nampally Station Rd., 500 001/ Tel. (040) 24744969 or 24607089/ iskcon.hyderabad@pamho.net

Imphal, Manipur — Hare Krishna Land, Airport Rd., 795 001/ Tel. (0385) 2455245 or 2455247 or 2455693/ manimandir@sancharnet.in

Indore, MP — ISKCON, Nipania, Indore/ Tel. 9300474043/ mahaman.acbsp@pamho.net

Jaipur, Rajasthan — ISKCON Road, Opp. Vijay Path, Mansarovar, Jaipur 302 020 (mail: ISKCON, 84/230, Sant Namdev Marg, Opp. K.V. No. 5, Mansarovar, Jaipur 302 020)/ Tel. (0414) 2782765 or 2781860/ jaipur@pamho.net

Jammu, J&K — Srila Prabhupada Ashram, c/o Shankar Charitable Trust, Shakti Nagar, Near AG Office/ Tel. (01991) 233047

Kolkata (Calcutta), WB — 3C Albert Rd., 700 017 (behind Minto Park, opp. Birla High School)/ Tel. (033) 3028-9258 or -9280/ iskcon.calcutta@pamho.net

• **Kurukshetra, Haryana** — 369 Gudri Muhalla, Main Bazaar, 132 118/ Tel. (01744) 234806

Lucknow, UP — 1 Ashok Nagar, Guru Govind Singh Marg, 226 018/ Tel. (0522) 223556 or 271551

• **Mayapur, WB** — ISKCON, Shree Mayapur Chandrodaya Mandir, Shree Mayapur Dham, Dist. Nadia, 741 313/ Tel. (03472) 245239, 245240, or 245233/ Fax: (03472) 245238/ mayapur.chandrodaya@pamho.net

• **Mumbai (Bombay), Maharashtra** — Hare Krishna Land, Juhu 400 049/ Tel. (022) 26206860/ Fax: (022) 26205214/ info@iskconmumbai.com; guest.house.bombay@pamho.net

• **Mumbai, Maharashtra** — 7 K. M. Munshi Marg, Chowpatty 400 007 / Tel. (022) 23665500/ Fax: (022) 23665555/ info@radhagopinath.com

Mumbai, Maharashtra — Shristhi Complex, Mira Rd. (E), opposite Royal College, Dist. Thane, 401 107/ Tel. (022) 28454667 or 28454672/ Fax: (022) 28454981/ jagjivan.gkg@pamho.net

Mysore, Karnataka — #31, 18th Cross, Jayanagar, 570 014/ Tel. (0821) 2500582 or 6567333/ mysore.iskcon@gmail.com

Nellore, AP — ISKCON City, Hare Krishna Rd., 524 004/ Tel. (0861) 2314577 or (092155) 36589/ sukadevaswami@gmail.com

• **New Delhi, UP** — Hare Krishna Hill, Sant Nagar Main Road, East

of Kailash, 110 065/ Tel. (011) 2623-5133, 4, 5, 6, 7/ Fax: (011) 2621-5421/ delhi@pamho.net; (Guesthouse) neel.sunder@pamho.net
• **New Delhi, UP** — 41/77, Punjabi Bagh (West), 110 026/ Tel. (011) 25222851 or 25227478 Noida, UP — A-5, Sector 33, opp. NTPC office, Noida 201 301/ Tel. (0120) 2506211/ vraja.bhakti.vilas.lok@pamho.net
Patna, Bihar — Arya Kumar Rd., Rajendra Nagar, 800 016/ Tel. (0612) 687637 or 685081/ Fax: (0612) 687635/ krishna.kripa.jps@pamho.net
Pune, Maharashtra — 4 Tarapoor Rd., Camp, 411 001/ Tel. (020) 26332328 or 26361855/ iyfpune@vsnl.com
Puri, Orissa — Bhakti Kuti, Swargadwar, 752 001/ Tel. (06752) 231440 Raipur, Chhatisgarh — Hare Krishna Land, Alopi Nagar, Opposite Maharshi Vidyalaya, Tatibandh, Raipur 492 001/ Tel. (0771) 5037555/ iskconraipur@yahoo.com
Secunderabad, AP — 27 St. John's Rd., 500 026/ Tel. (040) 780-5232/ Fax: (040) 814021
Silchar, Assam — Ambikapatti, Silchar, Dist. Cachar, 788 004/ Tel. (03842) 34615
Sri Rangam, TN — 103 Amma Mandapam Rd., Sri Rangam, Trichy 620 006/ Tel. (0431) 2433945/ iskcon_srirangam@yahoo.com.in
Surat, Gujarat — Rander Rd., Jahangirpura, 395 005/ Tel. (0261) 765891, 765516, or 773386/ surat@pamho.net
• **Thiruvananthapuram (Trivandrum), Kerala** — Hospital Rd., Thycaud, 695 014/ Tel. (0471) 2328197/ jsdasa@yahoo.co.in
• **Tirupati, AP** — K.T. Rd., Vinayaka Nagar, 517 507/ Tel. (0877) 2230114 or 2230009/ revati.raman.jps@pamho.net (guesthouse: iskcon_ashram@yahoo.co.in)
Udhampur, J&K — Srila Prabhupada Ashram, Srila Prabhupada Marg, Srila Prabhupada Nagar 182 101/ Tel. (01992) 270298/ info@iskconudhampur.com
Ujjain, MP — Hare Krishna Land, Bharatpuri, 456 010/ Tel. (0734) 2535000 or 3205000/ Fax: (0734) 2536000/ iskcon.ujjain@pamhho.net
Varanasi, UP — ISKCON, B 27/80 Durgakund Rd., Near Durgakund Police Station, Varanasi 221 010/ Tel. (0542) 246422 or 222617
• **Vrindavan, UP** — Krishna-Balaram Mandir, Bhaktivedanta Swami Marg, Raman Reti, Mathura Dist., 281 124/ Tel. & Fax: (0565) 2540728/ iskcon.vrindavan@pamho.net; (Guesthouse:) Tel. (0565) 2540022; ramamani@sancharnet.in

ADDITIONAL RESTAURANT

Kolkata, WB — Govinda's, ISKCON House, 22 Gurusaday Rd., 700 019/ Tel. (033) 24756922, 24749009

EUROPE (partial list)*

Amsterdam — Van Hilligaertstraat 17, 1072 JX/ Tel. +31 (020) 675-1404 or -1694/ Fax: +31 (020) 675-1405/ amsterdam@pamho.net
Barcelona — Plaza Reial 12, Entlo 2, 08002/ Tel. +34 93 302-5194/ templobcn@hotmail.com
Bergamo, Italy — Villaggio Hare Krishna (da Medolago strada per Terno d'Isola), 24040 Chignolo d'Isola (BG)/ Tel. +39 (035) 4940706
Budapest — Lehel Street 15–17, 1039 Budapest/ Tel. +36 (01) 391-0435/ Fax: (01) 397-5219/ nai@pamho.net
Copenhagen — Skjulhoj Alle 44, 2720 Vanlose, Copenhagen/ Tel. +45 4828 6446/ Fax: +45 4828 7331/ iskcon.denmark@pamho.net
Grödinge, Sweden — Radha-Krishna Temple, Korsnäs Gård, 14792 Grödinge, Tel.+46 (08) 53029800/ Fax: +46 (08) 53025062 / bmd@pamho.net
Helsinki — Ruoholahdenkatu 24 D (III krs) 00180/ Tel. +358 (9) 694-9879 or -9837
• **Lisbon** — Rua Dona Estefânia, 91 R/C 1000 Lisboa/ Tel. & fax: +351(01) 314-0314 or 352-0038
Madrid — Espíritu Santo 19, 28004 Madrid/ Tel. +34 91 521-3096
Paris — 35 Rue Docteur Jean Vaquier, 93160 Noisy le Grand/ Tel. & fax: +33 (01) 4303-0951/ param.gati.swami@pamho.net
Prague — Jilova 290, Prague 5 - Zlicin 155 21/ Tel. +42 (02) 5795-0391/ info@harekrsna.cz
• **Radhadesh, Belgium** — Chateau de Petite Somme, 6940 Septon-Durbuy/ Tel. +32 (086) 322926 (restaurant: 321421)/ Fax: +32 (086) 322929/ radhadesh@pamho.net
• **Rome** — Govinda Centro Hare Krsna, via di Santa Maria del Pianto 16, 00186/ Tel. +39 (06) 68891540/ govinda.roma@harekrsna.it
• **Stockholm** — Fridhemsgatan 22, 11240/ Tel. +46 (08) 654-9002/ Fax: +46 (08) 650-881; Restaurant: Tel. & fax: +46 (08) 654-9004/ lokanatha@hotmail.com
Warsaw — Mysiadlo k. Warszawy, 05-500 Piaseczno, ul. Zakret 11/ Tel. +48 (022) 750-7797 or -8247/ Fax: +48 (022) 750-8249/ kryszna@post.pl
Zürich — Bergstrasse 54, 8030/ Tel. +41 (01) 262-3388/ Fax: +41 (01) 262-3114/ kgs@pamho.net

RURAL COMMUNITIES

France (La Nouvelle Mayapura) — Domaine d'Oublaisse, 36360, Lucay le Mâle/ Tel. +33 (02) 5440-2395/ Fax: +33 (02) 5440-2823/ oublaise@free.fr
Germany (Simhachalam) — Zielberg 20, 94118 Jandelsbrunn/ Tel. +49 (08583) 316/ info@simhachalam.de
Hungary (New Vraja-dhama) — Krisna-völgy, 8699 Somogyvamos, Fö u, 38/ Tel. & fax: +36 (085) 540-002 or 340-185/ info@krisnavolgy.hu
Italy (Villa Vrindavan) — Via Scopeti 108, 50026 San Casciano in Val di Pesa (FL)/ Tel. +39 (055) 820054/ Fax: +39 (055) 828470/ isvaripriya@libero.it
Spain (New Vraja Mandala) — (Santa Clara) Brihuega, Guadalajara/ Tel. +34 949 280436

ADDITIONAL RESTAURANTS

Barcelona — Restaurante Govinda, Plaza de la Villa de Madrid 4–5, 08002/ Tel. +34 (93) 318-7729
Copenhagen — Govinda's, Nørre Farimagsgade 82, DK-1364 Kbh K/ Tel. +45 3333 7444
Milan — Govinda's, Via Valpetrosa 5, 20123/ Tel. +39 (02) 862417
Oslo — Krishna's Cuisine, Kirkeveien 59B, 0364/ Tel. +47 (02) 260-6250
Zürich — Govinda Veda-Kultur, Preyergrasse 16, 8001/ Tel. & fax: +41 (01) 251-8859/ info@govinda-shop.ch

CIS (partial list)*

Kiev — 16, Zorany per., 04078/ Tel. +380 (044) 433-8312, or 434-7028 or -5533
Moscow — 8/3, Khoroshevskoye sh. (mail: P.O. Box 69), 125284/ Tel. +7 (095) 255-6711/ Tel. & fax: +7 (095) 945-3317

ASIA (partial list)*

Bangkok, Thailand — Soi3, Tanon Itsarapap, Toonburi/ Tel. +66 (02) 9445346 or (081) 4455401 or (089) 7810623/ swami.bvv.narasimha@pamho.net
Dhaka, Bangladesh — 5 Chandra Mohon Basak St., Banagram,1203/ Tel. +880 (02) 236249/ Fax: (02) 837287/ iskcon_bangladesh@yahoo.com
Hong Kong — 6/F Oceanview Court, 27 Chatham Road South (mail: P.O. Box 98919)/ Tel. +852 (2) 739-6818/ Fax: +852 (2) 724-2186/ iskcon.hong.kong@pamho.net
Jakarta, Indonesia — Yayasan Radha-Govinda, P.O. Box 2694, Jakarta Pusat 10001/ Tel. +62 (021) 489-9646/ matsyads@bogor.wasantara.net.id

Katmandu, Nepal — Budhanilkantha (mail: GPO Box 3520)/ Tel. +977 (01) 373790 or 373786/ Fax: +977 (01) 372976 (Attn: ISKCON)/ iskcon@wlink.com.np
Kuala Lumpur, Malaysia — Lot 9901, Jalan Awan Jawa, Taman Yarl, 58200 Kuala Lumpur/ Tel. +60 (3) 7980-7355/ Fax: +60 (3) 7987-9901/ president@iskconkl.com
Manila, Philippines — Radha-Madhava Center, #9105 Banuyo St., San Antonio village, Makati City/ Tel. +63 (02) 8963357; Tel. & fax: +63 (02) 8901947/ iskconmanila@yahoo.com
Myitkyina, Myanmar — ISKCON Sri Jagannath Temple, Bogyoke Street, Shansu Taung, Myitkyina, Kachin State/ mahanadi@mptmail.net.mm
Tai Pei City, Taiwan — Ting Zhou Rd. Section 3, No. 192, 4F, Tai Pei City 100/ Tel. +886 (02) 2365-8641/ dayal.nitai.tkg@pamho.net
Tokyo, Japan — Subaru 1F, 4-19-6 Kamitakada, Nakano-ku, Tokyo 164-0002/ Tel. +81 (03) 5343- 9147 or (090) 6544-9284/ Fax: +81 (03) 5343-3812/ damodara@krishna.jp

LATIN AMERICA (partial list)*

Buenos Aires, Argentina — Centro Bhaktivedanta, Andonaegui 2054, Villa Urquiza, CP 1431/ Tel. +54 (01) 523-4232/ Fax: +54 (01) 523-8085/ iskcon-ba@gopalnet.com
Caracas, Venezuela — Av. Los Proceres (con Calle Marquez del Toro), San Bernardino/ Tel. +58 (212) 550-1818
Guayaquil, Ecuador — 6 de Marzo 226 and V. M. Rendon/ Tel. +593 (04) 308412 or 309420/ Fax: +564 302108/ gurumani@gu.pro.ec
• **Lima, Peru** — Schell 634 Miraflores/ Tel. +51 (014) 444-2871
Mexico City, Mexico — Tiburcio Montiel 45, Colonia San Miguel, Chapultepec D.F., 11850/ Tel. +52 (55) 5273-1953/ Fax: +52 (55) 52725944
Rio de Janeiro, Brazil — Rua Vilhena de Morais, 309, Barra da Tijuca, 22793-140/ Tel. +55 (021) 2491-1887/ sergio.carvalho@pobox.com
San Salvador, El Salvador — Calle Chiltiupan #39, Ciudad Merliot, Nueva San Salvador (mail: A.P. 1506)/ Tel. +503 2278-7613/ Fax: +503 2229-1472/ tulasikrishnadas@yahoo.com
São Paulo, Brazil — Rua do Paraiso, 694, 04103-000/Tel. +55 (011) 326-0975/ communicacaomandir@grupos.com.br
West Coast Demerara, Guyana — Sri Gaura Nitai Ashirvad Mandir, Lot "B," Nauville Flanders (Crane Old Road), West Coast Demerara/ Tel. +592 254 0494/ iskcon.guyana@yahoo.com

AFRICA (partial list)*

Accra, Ghana — Samsam Rd., Off Accra-Nsawam Hwy., Medie, Accra North (mail: P.O. Box 11686)/ Tel. & fax +233 (021) 229988/ srivas_bts@yahoo.co.in
Cape Town, South Africa — 17 St. Andrews Rd., Rondebosch 7700/ Tel. +27 (021) 6861179/ Fax: +27 (021) 686-8233/ cape.town@pamho.net
• **Durban, South Africa** — 50 Bhaktivedanta Swami Circle, Unit 5 (mail: P.O. Box 56003), Chatsworth, 4030/ Tel. +27 (031) 403-3328/ Fax: +27 (031) 403-4429/ iskcon.durban@pamho.net
Johannesburg, South Africa — 7971 Capricorn Ave. (entrance on Nirvana Drive East), Ext. 9, Lenasia (mail: P.O. Box 926, Lenasia 1820)/ Tel. +27 (011) 854-1975 or 7969/ iskconjh@iafrica.com
Lagos, Nigeria — 12, Gani Williams Close, off Osolo Way, Ajao Estate, International Airport Rd. (mail: P.O. Box 8793, Marina)/ Tel. +234 (01) 7744926 or 7928906/ bdds.bts@pamho.net
Mombasa, Kenya — Hare Krishna House, Sauti Ya Kenya and Kisumu Rds. (mail: P.O. Box 82224, Mombasa)/ Tel. +254 (011) 312248
Nairobi, Kenya — Muhuroni Close, off West Nagara Rd. (mail: P.O. Box 28946)/ Tel. +254 (203) 744365/ Fax: +254 (203) 740957/ iskcon_nairobi@yahoo.com
• **Phoenix, Mauritius** — Hare Krishna Land, Pont Fer (mail: P.O. Box 108, Quartre Bornes)/ Tel. +230 696-5804/ Fax: +230 696-8576/ iskcon.hkl@intnet.mu
Port Harcourt, Nigeria — Umuebule 11, 2nd tarred road, Etche (mail: P.O. Box 4429, Trans Amadi)/ Tel. +234 08033215096/ canakyaus@yahoo.com
Pretoria, South Africa — 1189 Church St., Hatfield, 0083 (mail: P.O. Box 14077, Hatfield, 0028)/ Tel. & fax: +27 (12) 342-6216/ iskconpt@global.co.za

RURAL COMMUNITY

Mauritius (ISKCON Vedic Farm) — Hare Krishna Rd., Vrindaban/ Tel. +230 418-3185 or 418-3955/ Fax: +230 418-6470

***The full list is always available at Krishna.com, where it also includes Krishna conscious gatherings.**